Skin Deep

Skin Deep

The Making of a Plastic Surgeon

Donald T. Moynihan, M.D.
and Shirley Hartman

LITTLE, BROWN AND COMPANY

BOSTON   TORONTO

FIRST EDITION

Library of Congress Cataloging in Publication Data
Moynihan, Donald T
  Scapel.

  1. Moynihan, Donald T. 2. Plastic surgeons —
California — Biography. 3. Residents (Medicine) —
California — Biography. I. Hartman, Shirley,
joint author. II. Title.
RD27.35.M68A33   617'.95'00924 [B]   79–10552
ISBN 0–316–58700–1

BP

Designed by D. Christine Benders

*Published simultaneously in Canada
by Little, Brown & Company (Canada) Limited*

PRINTED IN THE UNITED STATES OF AMERICA

"Beauty is only skin
deep — but ugly goes
all the way to bone."

Author's Note

PLASTIC SURGERY IS ONE of the youngest medical specialties. It has been considered by some to be a bastard field because it is directed to no one particular area, organ, or disease. The skin and all it covers — the human body from head to toe — is included in the domain of the plastic surgeon. Little by little, people are beginning to realize that they no longer have to live with correctable problems of appearance . . . nor do they necessarily have to suffer the disfiguring after-effects of wounds and injuries and some illnesses. The bastard has now found its legitimacy.

This is the story of my plastic surgery training. Everything discussed in this book actually happened.

The aura of secrecy that until recently has been demanded by the medical profession is gone — there is nothing wrong with the consumers of medical care gaining insight and knowledge about their doctors.

The confidentiality regarding their medical affairs that is the right of individuals, however, is quite another thing. It must be safeguarded. Consequently, the name and locale of the hospital and the identities of patients, doctors, and staff members have been altered to protect their privacy.

Donald T. Moynihan, M.D.

Skin Deep

Chapter One

8:47 A.M. I STRAIGHTENED MY SHOULDERS, then my starched tunic. It was the very first day of my plastic surgery residency at University Hospital in California, and I was determined to make a good impression. Having deliberately made ward rounds early, I'd been fidgeting in my tiny office since shortly after eight, waiting for the clinic to open. Outpatient hours were scheduled from nine until noon on Tuesdays, and from one until three in the afternoon on Thursdays.

Plastic surgery clinics in university hospitals are set up to deliver medical care and to insure an adequate flow of teaching cases. In clinics, medical care is available at costs substantially lower — perhaps fifty percent less — than if the patient were going to a private surgeon. At University Hospital we dealt basically with two types of case: cosmetic surgery and trauma or congenital deformities. For cosmetic surgery in the clinic, we got neither the affluent nor the indigent. A well-to-do patient will seek out a private surgeon for a face-lift or breast implant, and since cosmetic surgery is not covered by medical insurance, the extremely poor usually forgo it entirely. So middle-class people who desired cosmetic surgery and were concerned with out-of-pocket costs were numerous. Depending on their ability to pay, a three-thousand-dollar face-lift, for instance, would cost about a thousand dollars. It was carefully explained to each patient that a resident in training would be doing part of the surgery, well supervised by one of the staff plastic surgeons. Where trauma or congenital deformities were involved, it was already well known that we employed the latest techniques and accepted all types of insurance coverage. The clinic was popular, and I knew the waiting room was already crammed with patients. I wondered if any of them was as anxious as I was.

I counted the seconds as the clock's hands crept forward, and at nine on the dot sauntered casually to Miss Farrell's desk, where the charts were stacked, arranged in the order of the patients' actual arrival. There were no appointments at the Plastic Surgery Outpatient Clinic; it was strictly first come, first served.

My appearance caused twenty heads to turn, and as twenty pairs of eyes followed my progress, I felt the reverence for that white coat like a physical thing. If you can believe the Gallup Polls, Americans have a respect for physicians second only to that for the Justices of the U.S. Supreme Court. One of my psychiatry professors in medical school had said, "The reason why you, as future doctors, will be held in inordinate awe, and will be overpaid, is because there is nothing people value more than their own bodies. They will transfer that respect to you, the healer of their bodies." Maybe so. But any conceit such recollections conjured up was quickly punctured by Miss Farrell. As I approached the receptionist with a cheery "Good morning," she pointedly ignored me. To her, anyone except Dr. Lawrence M. Parmenter was almost invisible. She viewed residents as legs to run to assist him, hands to pick up the charts, automatons who might possibly take some of the load from the great man's shoulders.

Besides acting as receptionist at the Outpatient Clinic, Miss Farrell was the personal secretary, assistant, Mother Superior, confidante, and second self of Dr. Parmenter, the Chief of the Plastic Surgery Department at University Hospital. A year or so away from forty, she wore her hair stylishly short, and her inevitable suits were expensive, conservative, and serviceable. Her face, always a mask of efficiency unless the presence of Dr. Parmenter inspired animation, was not unattractive, but her general aspect was forbidding.

I would not let her spoil my morning. I picked up the top chart and read aloud, "Miss Celeste Bigliani?" and looked about expectantly. A young girl rose immediately, and I started to lead her into one of the two examining rooms before I was aware that she was flanked on one side by an older woman, while a tall sad-looking man doggedly trailed a few steps behind us.

5

Miss Farrell looked up with a frown. "Only the patient, please, in the examining room," she snapped.

The older woman missed not a step. "I am her mama," she pronounced. I saw Miss Farrell gird herself for battle, caught her glance, and almost imperceptibly shook my head. I wanted no problems with my very first patient; besides, there was childish satisfaction in thwarting Miss Farrell's ordained protocol. It was a satisfaction I would soon regret.

"Good morning. I'm Dr. Moynihan, one of the plastic surgeons here. Would you sit down, please," I said to the patient, indicating the examining table. I waited until she had settled herself, using the interval to glance at the chart. Twenty-four, single. "Would you like to tell me about your problem?" I smiled at her.

"She has no problem!" Mama answered before the girl could speak.

Ignoring her, the daughter looked at me. "My nose," she began softly.

Mama's voice rose an octave. "Her nose! She should be proud! Right from her papa she got it. Tell her, doctor! There's nothing wrong with her nose. Her brother, Roberto — does it bother him? It runs in the family. For generations —"

"Mrs. Bigliani —" I interrupted.

"The g is silent." These were the first words that the tall, hook-nosed man accompanying them had uttered. "Billy-ani," her father corrected me gently.

The mother nodded, "A famous name," she said proudly. "Descended from counts. In Rome." She got

6

back to the matter at hand, addressing her daughter. "God will punish you," she whispered, crossing herself. "You're tampering with His doing. You're a beautiful girl."

.And indeed she was. Long, almost black, silky hair. A fine complexion. I sidled to the left for a profile view under the harsh examining light. A beautiful girl — full-face. But from the side, her prominently hooked nose made her look like a witch.

"I'm through arguing," the girl said. "On a boy, maybe it isn't so bad. But all my life I've hated my nose. I pass windows and I force myself not to look at the reflection. You know, doctor, when I was graduating from high school, someone told me that the photographer insisted on taking profile portraits for the yearbook — so I just didn't show up." The strength of her voice increased. "From the time I was eighteen, I've worked. I've saved every penny I could. Now I can afford to have it fixed — if it's possible."

"It's possible," I said.

Mama Bigliani groaned and glared at me. "You're young!"

"Over thirty," I countered, "and married." Why was I being so defensive?

"How do we know you know what you're doing?" she demanded.

I sighed. The sigh would have been louder if I'd had any conception of how often I would be forced to defend my youthful appearance and explain the seemingly mysterious field in which I specialized.

7

"Mrs. Bigliani," I said, careful to pronounce the name correctly, "I am a qualified surgeon. I have spent four years in college, four years in medical school, one year of internship, four years in general surgery residency, and I'm the senior plastic surgery resident here at University Hospital." I neglected to mention that I was the *only* plastic surgery resident. "Thirteen years of training," I emphasized. As she started to interrupt, I gazed at my patient. She was of age, and psychologically was a good candidate for the operation. She wanted the cosmetic improvement for no one's benefit except her own, and it was obvious that her decision was not a spur-of-the-moment one.

Mama was beginning to bug me, and I opted for drastic action.

"You'll both have to wait outside while I examine the patient," I said authoritatively. Never again would I question a dictum from Miss Farrell. Before they could argue, I herded Mr. and Mrs. Bigliani out, firmly closing the door on their heels. Then I turned back to my patient.

"What we're talking about is known as rhinoplasty," I explained, "and I can assure you that considerable improvement is possible." The grateful expression on her face was satisfying. Nose jobs have often been the subject of jokes. Even other doctors sometimes chide plastic surgeons about this so-called frivolous surgery. What's frivolous about correcting a serious defect in appearance that can negatively affect social life and personality? All I can say is, if you're the one with a honker for a nose, it's not so funny.

8

I've always made it a practice to explain the entire procedure thoroughly to a prospective patient, taking care not to minimize the discomfort or the possible complications. Many candidates approach plastic surgery as casually as one might make an appointment with a hairdresser. But surgery is surgery. The risk is always there. So I took a deep breath.

"Rhinoplasty is a delicate procedure," I began, "but the likelihood of complications is pretty low. The most common one is excessive bleeding, but that can be dealt with by repacking. Infection is very unusual, though it can happen. Antibiotics usually clear it up." She nodded her understanding, and I went on. "Now, for the actual procedure. In your case, it will involve the shaving of the bone from the bridge of your nose to get rid of the prominent hump, the removal of some cartilage from the tip, and fracturing the bones and pushing them inward to narrow the shape. Then your nose will be taped and splinted in its new form."

She blinked. "It sounds . . . interesting."

"Very little pain, though," I assured her. "You'll be awake but heavily sedated. We'll use a local anesthetic. And we'll want you in the hospital the day before surgery for lab work and blood tests."

I was aware that some cosmetic surgeons did this procedure in their offices, but hospitalization for all plastic surgery was routine policy at our medical institution.

"No scars?" Miss Bigliani asked anxiously.

I shook my head. "All done internally. If we have to tuck in or remove any excess skin, it will be done at the

9

side of the nostrils, in the natural lines, where it won't show."

She nodded her understanding. "Will you wait here for a moment?" I asked. "I'll be right back."

The Plastic Surgery Outpatient Clinic was shaped like a horizontal H. One leg of the H was the big rectangular waiting room–reception area. The narrow connecting passage housed the two clinic examining rooms, with small, utilitarian cubbyholes in back of each for the residents. Across the rear swept Dr. Parmenter's office, with an attractive waiting area and a separate examining room for his private patients. Next to these were the much smaller and Spartan quarters of Dr. Alfred Burke, Parmenter's junior associate.

As I have mentioned, I was the only plastic surgery resident at the hospital. But because of the number of patients and since it was a teaching institution, there was always another young doctor, serving his general surgery residency, who was assigned to work with us for two months. When he left, another surgeon in training would take his place. Since these were first-year residents, they did little more than take down the patient's history, do a cursory examination, and determine, if they could, the problem. At that point, they would reduce the lengthy and often rambling dialogue of the patient to a succinct medical report for Dr. Parmenter or Dr. Burke, saving considerable time. Then the Chief of the Plastic Surgery Department or his associate examined the patient, diagnosed, and specified treatment or surgery. Having four years' ad-

ditional experience, I had been granted more leeway.
Unless an unusually complex procedure was involved,
I had authority to make diagnoses and schedule the
patient for admittance on my own.

I was well aware that Celeste Bigliani's case was an
uncomplicated one, but either because it was my first
patient or because her parents had intimidated me, I
longed for a confirmation of my judgment. As I headed
for Dr. Parmenter's office, I met Dr. Bob Sutton, the
resident currently assigned to Plastic Surgery, coming
in the opposite direction.

"If you're looking for Parmenter, he hasn't come in
yet," Bob said. "And as far as Burke's concerned, forget
it. He's temporarily . . . unavailable."

I couldn't suppress a chuckle. Almost everyone in
the hospital was aware of Dr. Burke's ritualistic and
unvaried routine. Precisely fifteen minutes after he
arrived, he bolted himself inside a bathroom for exactly one half hour. Those thirty minutes were sacro-
sanct. Even Miss Farrell held his calls, important and
unimportant, not daring to buzz him for any reason. I
remember once hearing Dr. Neal Crenshaw, Chief of
General Surgery at the hospital, kidding him about
it.

"Christ, Al," he'd said, "can't you crap on your own
time?"

"I eat here, the crummy food digests here, so why in
the hell shouldn't I —" Burke had plodded away instead of completing the statement. A charmer he
wasn't.

11

"So he's in the can," I said to Bob. "Tough shit." We both broke up at the unintended pun before I headed back to Miss Bigliani. I'd have to do as I should have done in the first place — rely on my own experience and judgment. I knew Parmenter would concur.

Bob's words stopped me momentarily. "Jesus," he said plaintively, "what am I supposed to do with my patient? I don't know anything about —"

"Improvise," I interrupted. "Just keep talking and examining until you hear the flush."

Miss Bigliani was sitting quietly. "All right," I said, "whenever you want to go ahead with the surgery, just call Miss Farrell and she'll make admission arrangements."

"I want to have it done right away," she said, getting to her feet.

"Fine. Just tell the receptionist. She'll let you know when a bed will be available. Oh, and be sure to stop at the medical photographer's office before you leave. It's on the second floor."

"Photographer?" Miss Bigliani repeated warily.

"Yep," I said firmly, "full face, a three-quarter shot, and a profile, too. It's policy here to have 'before and after' photographs of all cases. No exceptions. Look," I continued reassuringly, "they'll be part of your medical records. Privileged information. No one will ever see them but the staff." It didn't seem pertinent to explain that one of the reasons for that procedure was the protection it provided the hospital and staff against possible malpractice suits. I preferred to remind myself that the photos were valuable teaching aids that could be used at future medical conferences. And often the "before" photographs were invaluable as guides during the actual surgical procedure. Resigned, she nodded and left.

As I started to follow her out to summon the next patient, I noticed Bob Sutton still nervously pacing up and down the hallway.

"Lord, Don," he groaned, "I've got a seventeen-year-old kid in there with a facial injury — and I don't know what to do. Damn Burke." He paused. "If I examine that boy one more time, he's going to think I'm a queer."

"Do you want me to take a look?" I offered.

"God, yes."

"Dr. Moynihan, this is Bernie Schweig," Bob said as I entered the examining room. The big burly kid perched on the examining table listened alertly as Bob filled me in. Six weeks ago Bernie had galloped into a goalpost during a football game. He hadn't even realized his cheekbone was fractured until the depression and slight asymmetry of his face had not improved. About two weeks later, he'd been operated on at another hospital, and since the surgeons there had been unable to reduce the fracture — to move the bone back into its original position — they had suggested he see us.

I checked the report of the referring surgeon attached to the chart. The approach used had been an incision through the outer portion of the right eyebrow so there would be no visible scar. A long, thin metal instrument called an elevator had then been inserted and positioned under the fractured cheekbone. The procedure had been to pull up on the elevator and move the bone back into its normal place. But by the time young Bernie had sought medical attention, the bone had partially healed and couldn't be dislodged. The surgeon who had signed the report had a good reputation, and I instinctively felt that every possible repair effort had already been exerted.

"I think we'd better get Dr. Burke to take a look," I said to Bob. Once he had left, Bernie Schweig squirmed uncomfortably for a moment.

"Doc, can I talk to you?"

"Sure. But about the cheekbone, you waited too long. I'm not sure there's anything we can do. . . ."

"I don't care. I only came because my mom insisted." He continued fidgeting.

"What's bothering you, Bernie?"

His voice dropped to a whisper, and he glanced about, afraid he might be overheard. "Well, I've been fooling around with a couple of girls lately — and I think there's something wrong with me." The last phrase was almost inaudible.

"You mean you can't get an erection?" He lowered his eyes. "You can't get it up?"

"No," he mumbled, "no problem there. It's just — it's just — well, I don't come off."

I suppose it is an indictment of the physician's current fetish for specialization, but my immediate impulse was to refer his ejaculation problem to urology, with the recommendation that if their findings were negative, he see one of the hospital's psychiatrists. It was only because Dr. Sutton had not yet returned with the elusive Dr. Burke that I felt compelled to go on with the conversation.

Little by little, I wormed the facts from him. Facing me was an only child, the product of a strict religious upbringing. He'd never masturbated in his life, and intercourse was a recent experience — therefore, we couldn't compare his present performance with past ones to determine if there'd been a change.

Had he discussed the problem with his father? God, no!! His coach? Maybe some of the other boys?

"I couldn't," he said utterly abashed. "I just couldn't do that."

Finally I asked for an exact description of what happened at the end of intercourse and he described what, to me, seemed a normal ejaculation. The light finally dawned. He didn't know what normal sexual function was supposed to be like. He evidently thought that sperm should take off like a rocket.

"What you've experienced is normal, Bernie," I reassured him. "Absolutely normal. Like that song by Peggy Lee — that's all there is." Delight and relief washed over his face, and he was still grinning when Dr. Sutton returned, followed by Dr. Parmenter.

Bob had obviously informed the Chief of Plastic Surgery of the problem, for Dr. Parmenter wasted no time. A quick look, a minute of probing the facial area with his fingers, a glance at the X-rays, and he shook his head.

"Sorry, son. Nothing we can do." His warm smile and fleeting sympathetic clasp of the boy's shoulder softened the crisp words.

"That's all right, sir. Thank you," Bernie called as Parmenter hurried out. Then the patient shook hands with me, and left, a happy young man.

When I called out the name Patricia Niles, a very attractive sixteen-year-old black girl got up and followed me into the examining room. I could not see anything the matter with her until she removed the colorful scarf from her head. She had pierced her own ears three years ago — and had developed complications. Keloids, greatly enlarged scars, had formed. These can occur in any person, but people with dark pigmentation are much more likely to be plagued by them. Poor Patty. She had masses of scar tissue the size of marbles dangling from each earlobe. I assured her it was a simple matter to correct. We could cut out the keloid and a small area surrounding it, then stitch the skin edges at the back of the ear where it wouldn't show. An injection of a steroid in the new scar would help insure normal healing. She was scheduled for surgery on Monday, when we did minor operations that could be done under local anesthesia.

I followed Patty out and was about to pick up the next chart, when Miss Farrell deigned to look up.

"Dr. Parmenter wants to talk to you before he leaves for lunch, Dr. Moynihan. You'd better see him now.

Dr. Sutton can continue with the patients." It was not a suggestion, it was a command.

I bristled at her tone, but only for a moment. I owed a lot to Dr. Parmenter. From the time I was seven years old, I'd known I had to be a doctor. It was strange, because no one else in my family is an M.D. Practically everybody is a lawyer. My father is a judge and law professor who has written a textbook used in universities throughout the country. My brother, Neil, is a lawyer practicing in Boston and his wife is going to law school. Even my sister, Anne, is a paralegal, and married to an attorney, yet. But medicine was for me. I just knew it. And during my junior year at medical school, I'd made the big decision. I decided I wanted to be in a field that allowed direct therapy for curable problems. Surgery offered this, and gave the satisfaction of immediate results — unlike, say, psychiatry, where I would never stop wondering if any permanent improvement was ever effected. Or internal medicine, where many of the problems were chronic and, with rare exceptions, the treatment was supportive rather than curative. Yes, I would be a surgeon!

In his senior year, each would-be doctor chooses a number of hospitals throughout the country at which he might like to serve his internship, and he files formal applications. A face-to-face interview is scheduled with each institution that expresses interest, a costly procedure for the student, incidentally, since he must pay his own traveling expenses. Then he lists his preferences in order and forwards his choices to a computerized process known as the Intern Matching Program. Basing their decisions on the personal interviews, augmented by grades, personalities, and recommendations from the medical schools, the various hospitals respond by forwarding to the computer center a list of intern candidates in the order of *their* preference. Then, on a specified day, after the computers have done their work, every senior medical student is handed a sealed letter telling him the results: his highest listed preference matched with the hospital that has requested him. Inside that one envelope is a career decision that will affect his future life, his potential income, that even dictates where he will live. Tearing open the sealed flap can be compared only to exploring the interior of a celestial fortune cookie straight from God.

Like every medical student, I had listed a wide range of hospitals, ending up with a remote one in Canada. I wasn't taking any chances! But my first choice had been University Hospital and, praise the Lord, they wanted me. So, when I graduated, I headed there for my internship, and stayed on for my four years of general surgery residency.

Late one night during my third year at the hospital, at the end of a hectic day, I happened to be on the elevator when it stopped at the emergency ward floor. A girl of about twelve, suffering severe facial lacerations from an automobile accident, had been wheeled in on a stretcher. She was being taken to the operating room by the hospital's plastic surgeon, Dr. Lawrence

Parmenter. I was dead tired, practically out on my feet, but something about the girl's injuries and the tall, confident man standing beside her mesmerized me. I found myself asking if I could assist him during the operation. At the time, there were no interns or residents officially assigned to the Plastic Surgery service, and the lateness of the hour made other help unavailable, so he was delighted to have me.

The girl's face was a horrible mess. From her gums to her eyes, the skin and muscles of the cheeks were torn away from the underlying bones. Her lips were shredded in a number of places, and loose flaps of skin hung in different directions. I helped Dr. Parmenter clean each wound with sterile soap and water, and watched with awe as he meticulously sutured the tissue back into place. He closed the lacerations with very fine stitches, cutting away dead skin with precision instruments. He put the skin flaps back into place and tacked them down with great care. By five A.M., a face that four hours before had been a disaster had undergone a metamorphosis, and now, considering the injuries, looked relatively normal.

Next to this technique, all other operations I had witnessed seemed gross. It was at that precise moment that I decided to become a plastic surgeon.

The man who could help me attain my goal was Dr. Parmenter. Undeniably a handsome man, he stood six feet tall, with dark brown curly hair, sparkling blue eyes, and a smile that revealed teeth so white and even that I've only seen their likes in the mouth of a merry-go-round horse. And he was a charmer. His patients adored him, not only because he was a topnotch plastic surgeon, but he was affable, caring and sensitive to their needs. He was equally popular among his own; his colleagues sought his advice and friendship. He was only forty years old and had married money. He and his wife belonged to the best clubs, resided in the most elegant suburb, and entertained lavishly. His car was the flashiest in the doctors' parking area; his clothes were specially fashioned by the most expert tailors. Only one thing marred his utopian existence.

University Hospital was large, world-famous, and heavily endowed. As a teaching institution, it teemed with medical students and had departments in every conceivable field — urology, neurology, gynecology, internal medicine, pediatrics, psychiatry, ear, nose, and throat, orthopedics — you name it. The Chief of General Surgery was Dr. Neal Crenshaw, a crochety man pushing sixty. With numerous surgeons under his command, supported by no fewer than twenty surgical residents, he was one of the most powerful figures in the institution. Bearing the weight of his responsibility seriously, he was punctilious, testy, and negative, and saw himself as the watchdog of the entire hospital. But the greatest inequity, from Parmenter's viewpoint, was that this disparaging, jealous, acerbic man was officially over him. Dr. Lawrence Parmenter was only one of nine or ten staff surgeons on Dr. Crenshaw's service.

In a large teaching hospital, medical politics are, unfortunately, a way of life. If it appears unseemly that doctors aggressively compete with each other for cases, the fact remains that the go-for-the-jugular competition is very real. As I said, Dr. Parmenter was good, and every surgical case was a challenge. He liked nothing better than being handed an interesting and difficult procedure. Unfortunately, unlike any other specialty, there are virtually no patients that can be labeled as belonging exclusively to the field of plastic surgery. In his official position of power, aware of the many general surgery students, interns, and residents he had to train, while plastic surgery had none, Dr. Crenshaw persisted in assigning burn patients to his general surgeons, hand injuries to his Orthopedic Department, and neck cancers to the Ear, Nose and Throat Service.

Dr. Parmenter was an egotistical man. He watched what he considered *his* cases being doled out to his competitors. He tolerated it for a time. But in addition to being a competent surgeon, he was an expert infighter. Using his unbelievable charm, his guile, and his connections, Dr. Parmenter was somehow able to convince the Board of Directors to establish a Department of Plastic Surgery and a Plastic Surgery Clinic, with himself at the head. And, most important, they agreed that it would be autonomous, independent of the General Surgery Service. It was Dr. Parmenter's baby. The deal he negotiated is known in medical circles as "geographical full time" — in other words, he was obligated to spend a hundred percent of his working time at University Hospital for a stipulated salary of forty thousand dollars a year. For that, he would run the plastic surgery department and assist in the teaching of resident doctors, rotating interns, and medical students. He would lecture and lend his name to hospital activities. However, he was also allowed to have private patients, who would be individually billed, and this easily netted him an additional sixty thousand. The hospital equipped and supplied his office and examining rooms, and paid his secretary. Teaching hospitals are willing to make concessions and to pay handsomely to lure top medical talent to head their departments, for the quality of training depends on the expertise of the men at the top. Dr. Parmenter was aware that the title of Chief of Plastic Surgery at one of the world's foremost teaching institutions brought with it tremendous status and respect. Now, assured of a high standing and an adequate flow of patients — and having everything else — Dr. Parmenter found his life complete.

The Chief of the new Department of Plastic Surgery was a superb medical technician — and perhaps the world's lousiest administrator. To his credit, Dr. Parmenter recognized his failing. He quickly hired Roberta Farrell and delegated all administrative tasks and details to her. She ran his department smoothly and was readily accessible to solve any problem. It was rumored that Parmenter had pressured the hospital into paying her nearly $20,000 a year, considerably more than any resident earned. That knowledge, and her abrasive personality, did not endear her to the staff. Yet, on the one day when she was sick, chaos struck the department. Parmenter managed to schedule three operations for exactly the same time, fouled up his dictating equipment, and missed an important luncheon date to boot. Admittedly, Miss Farrell was a bitch — but worth every cent he paid her.

All of this had happened over a year ago — when I was beginning my final year of general surgery residency. In the interim, the volume of work had necessitated the hiring of a second plastic surgeon, Dr. Alfred Burke. Just out of training, Dr. Burke was about thirty-three years old, with sandy hair carefully combed and sprayed into a sweeping fringe over his forehead. Professionally, he was competent, but not exceptional. It was obvious that he viewed his current position as a postgrad training ground, a stepping stone to establishing his private practice. Paid $25,000 a year, and not permitted private patients, this dour and graceless man (and his family) had to live frugally in order to save enough money to eventually equip and sustain his own office. The contrast between his penny-pinching existence and Dr. Parmenter's luxurious life-style made him resentful. Nor did it help that Dr. Parmenter consistently referred to Burke not by name, but as "my number two man."

On that particular Wednesday night when I had been allowed to assist Dr. Parmenter through the difficult emergency operation, he was seething over the fact that Dr. Burke had not been available to take the call.

"Nice job," I said afterward. Dr. Parmenter nodded

his thanks. I sensed that now was the time to pursue an idea that had been in my mind for months.

"Have you ever considered establishing a plastic surgery residency, Dr. Parmenter?"

I held my breath as his eyes narrowed at the prospect. He was fully aware of my love for the field and was sensitive enough to suspect my motivation — that I was applying then and there. I was counting on the fact that he was sure of my loyalty. But there was more. Knowing his ego, I was hoping that the idea would appeal to him as a means of building up his blossoming department. And I wanted to work with him more than anything.

Within months, his charm prevailed — he had pulled the proper strings — and I found myself the first and only exclusive plastic surgery resident at University Hospital. Eighteen thousand a year, and all the work I could handle.

It was a coup for me. Medical students were fast recognizing plastic surgery as a fascinating and rewarding field. Eventually scientists will come up with cures for most of the illnesses that presently concern many specialists: cancer, high blood pressure, heart diseases. But injuries, congenital defects, pride, vanity, and concern with appearance will always be with us. Yet fewer than a hundred hospitals in the entire United States offer formal training in plastic surgery.

So, as I said, I owed Dr. Lawrence Parmenter a helluva lot. If he wanted to see me, I was already on my way.

I tapped at his door and entered. "Good morning, sir."

"Hi, Don." He gestured me to a chair. "Do me a favor. When you make afternoon rounds, pay special attention to the patient in 302. Be sure the history and physical are detailed and precise."

I nodded, strangely hurt. My histories and physicals were *always* detailed and precise. My bafflement showed, and he noticed.

"The kid's the current pet project of Mrs. Stardahl. You know who she is?"

"Yes."

Hell, yes. Who didn't? Socially prominent, immensely wealthy, her name linked with every charity drive in the city. Her cynical detractors whispered that Alicia Stardahl's philanthropy was overshadowed by her delight in seeing her photograph on the society pages almost every day; it was true that she retained a personal publicity man. But she was a dynamo of energy for any cause in which she believed, and she got results. With her at the helm, recent cancer drives, polio telethons, and multiple sclerosis benefits had attracted more dollars than ever before. For the past two years, she had been the president of University Hospital's Women's Auxiliary, and using her social connections with movie stars and studio heads, had managed to garner several important motion picture premieres, which benefited our institution by many hundreds of thousands of dollars. Occasionally, her charitable efforts were scaled to a one-to-one basis —

she would find a needy individual and devote her drive and unlimited money to helping that person. The reason for Parmenter's concern was obvious. It would be decidedly impolitic to annoy Mrs. Stardahl.

"What's the problem with the patient in 302?" I asked. "Is it a resident's case?"

Parmenter shook his head. "Since Alicia is involved, Dr. Burke and I will personally handle this one." He suddenly rose. "Got to get going or be late for a luncheon date. See you."

He was out the door before I realized he had not answered my original question.

I headed back to the Outpatient Clinic. Knowing that Dr. Parmenter was scheduled for an early lunch, Miss Farrell had leaned on Dr. Burke, and with Bob's assistance, he had taken care of all but one of the waiting patients.

This turned out to be a simple postoperative examination of a woman who'd suffered a facial cut and had undergone suturing about a week before. The laceration was healing nicely and when she left, the reception room was empty except for Miss Farrell, who was shuffling papers and getting her desk in order.

"I thought things went pretty well," I said, unconsciously searching for a compliment. "Didn't you?"

Her shrug was noncommittal. "Give my regards to the patient in 302," she said.

Chapter Two

I GULPED A GLASS OF MILK with a ham and Swiss cheese
sandwich, pondering on the meaning of Miss Farrell's parting shot. My speculations were broken off
when Agnes Tewksbury joined me.

Agnes was practically a charter member of University Hospital; for almost forty consecutive years she'd
been one of our telephone switchboard operators.
Approaching sixty-five, she certainly was not senile — I
guess "dithery" would be a better description. For instance, the hospital staff was still talking about an incident that had occurred several weeks ago. Her excited
voice had blasted through the paging system: "Code
blue! Code blue!" — followed by a click and utter silence. Now a Code Blue at our facility meant that a
patient was dying, and it was a signal for all available
medical help to respond at a dead run to help in resuscitation. The broadcast code is always followed by a

location: for example, "Code Blue — Emergency Room" or "Code Blue — Room 407," so time is not wasted in responding. After Mrs. T's cryptic announcement, you can imagine the consternation and pounding feet rushing for telephones to pinpoint where the crisis was.

Luckily there'd been two doctors near the room at the time a nurse discovered that a patient's heart had arrested, and they immediately started resuscitation. Help was right at hand, the patient lived, so no real harm was done. Agnes was reprimanded, of course, but it was a one-time oversight. Nobody's perfect — even in a hospital.

Agnes began picking at her peach and cottage cheese salad.

"How's it going?" she asked.

"Fine. Couldn't be better."

It was true. I was at the threshold of the last stage before becoming a full-fledged plastic surgeon. The course had been arduous, for the training required for plastic surgery is probably the longest of any medical specialty. It had been a busy, often difficult, thirteen years, beginning with my premedical training at Boston College. The premed group, approximately eighty students who shared the common goal of wanting to become physicians, were somewhat set apart from the general student body because most of their course of study was prearranged. It was heavy on required science, light on liberal arts, and very light on electives. Premedical students have little time for other campus activities because most of the science courses have laboratory sessions lasting into the late afternoon. Besides that, a lot of study time is involved. The premedical group at B.C. was also identifiable to some degree because of a prestige factor. It was recognized that we had one of the toughest programs offered. Everyone knew you had to work your tail off to get through premed.

That's exactly what I did, and in my senior year I found myself in the biggest struggle of all — getting into medical school. Medicine is a popular profession and there are far more applicants than spaces available. At the time I was applying, the ratio of applicants to openings was approximately four to one. The usual results are that most of the A students and somewhat more than fifty percent of the straight B students make it. Anyway, I was accepted and headed for St. Louis University Medical School.

The first week there was devoted to parties run by different fraternities to lure freshmen into their houses. The fraternity I joined has as its claim to fame the fact that the late Dr. Tom Dooley had been a brother some years before. When I arrived, one of the upper classmen escorted me to the rear of the structure, where he proudly displayed what remained of the back porch. He explained that Dr. Tom, who was a bit of a hell-raiser, had chopped the rest of it away with an ax during a jovial moment. But our fun and games ended abruptly the following week when classes started. The first year my study program permitted about four and a half hours' sleep a night. Classes and lab sessions at school ended around five P.M. I'd rush to the fraternity house for a quick twenty-minute dinner and before six I was back at the medical school library for a night of intensive studying until it closed at one A.M. Then I'd go across the street to take advantage of the University Hospital's library until three A.M.

Exam times were bad. Frequently before an examination I'd spend the entire night studying, not getting one minute's sleep. To keep awake, I'd often splash my face with cold water, and I kept a preset alarm clock beside me so that I would not miss the test, in case I dozed off. After an exam was over, I'd go back to the fraternity house and sleep. Boy, would I sleep. Once I slept eighteen straight hours, and when I finally woke up, I'd totally forgotten I'd taken the exam. Thinking I had missed it, I cussed out my roommate, Paul, for not waking me for the test. He didn't know what the hell I was talking about.

The first two years of medical school were pretty much the same: lectures, laboratory, study and exams. The second two years were considerably different and a great improvement, for they were spent in the hospital on various specialty services, working in the real world of medicine with live patients and their problems.

"I'd better be getting along." Agnes's words brought me back to the present with a start. I wondered if she'd resented my silence during lunch — or maybe, immersed in her own thoughts, she hadn't noticed.

"I'll walk you to the elevator," I said, hoping to

make amends. Then we parted and I headed for the nursing station of the third floor.

I picked up the chart for the patient in room 302. Timmy Rattigan, age seven. He had been born with terrible congenital defects — no eyes, no nose, and an enlarged head caused by hydrocephalus, a case that promised total misery from start to finish. According to the records, the child had spent the first three and a half months of his life in the County Hospital, for as soon as the parents found out what they had produced they had simply abandoned their son and disappeared. He had come to the attention of Mrs. Stardahl, and the hydrocephalus had been successfully treated at her expense. Once recovered from that, Timmy had been sent to the Freemont Orphanage, which was specially equipped to handle handicapped children. Since then, again at Mrs. Stardahl's urging, eyebrows had been implanted, but there were no eyeballs in the shallow sockets; there was no way Timmy could ever see. Then, inspired, Mrs. Stardahl had requested that we construct a nose for him, so that dark glasses would have a place to rest, glasses that would cover his empty eye sockets. That way, she said, he might at least appear in public without being looked at in horror. I reread that portion of the chart. If he were looked at with horror, he would never know. Was her kindness motivated by sympathy for the child, or sympathy for those who, like herself, might have to look at him?

I had my instructions — instructions right from the top — and I resolutely entered the room to examine him. I was greeted by the sight of a newly deposited pile of feces on the floor where he had relieved himself. Timmy was sitting in the corner, giggling and grunting.

I had seen deformed children before, but Timmy was the worst. I had the normal impulse to bolt from the room. But I have a special feeling for kids, and I began talking reassuringly to let him know I was there. He didn't even raise his head. I tried to pick him up to cuddle him, but he squirmed until I gave up. I noted on the chart, "Sensory input negligible." It was kinder than saying that he was grossly retarded. All I could do was check him carefully to make sure he was medically fit to undergo the scheduled surgery.

Once back at the nursing station, I completed writing my medical findings. That done, I reread the chart from start to finish — and came across a notation I had missed before. Four hours after birth, Timmy had gotten into difficulty ending in a cardiac arrest. Who's to say that it wasn't nature's way of dealing with this human disaster? There are many physicians who would argue with me, but in my opinion, the kindest thing would have been to let him die — but a gung-ho intern had worked frantically to resuscitate him. So Timmy survived — to face a life with which he was in no way fit to cope.

I finally managed to pull myself together and started making rounds, seeing the postoperative patients first. Even though their operations had been done before I joined the Plastic Surgery Department, they were now my responsibility. Normally, it didn't take long — a few new orders, removing some stitches, and double-checking on their condition. Everything was routine until one of the floor nurses sought me out.

"You'd better come take a look at Mrs. Vaughn, Dr. Moynihan. She's quite upset." I hurried after her.

Even before I entered the room, I could hear the moans and sobs coming from within. Mamie Vaughn, forty-four years of age, had undergone cosmetic eyelid surgery the day before. When I'd seen her earlier, she'd been groggy from sedation but had no complaints. Now she was crying hysterically.

"I'm blind," she whimpered. "Oh, dear God in heaven, I'm blind!"

"Take it easy," I murmured. "I'm right here. Try to calm down for a moment so I can take a look and see what this is all about."

I examined the eyes and the area surrounding them. The lids had the normal amount of swelling for this kind of surgery. The eyes themselves looked fine. I dug into my pocket for the visual acuity card that I'd learned to carry with me. It was an exact replica of the standard eye testing chart found in ophthalmologists' offices and drivers' license testing centers, scientifically scaled down so that when it was held fourteen inches from the eyes, the number of lines read gave a fairly accurate indication of vision. As Mrs. Vaughn spieled off line after line with no difficulty, I knew that all she needed was a liberal dose of reassurance. She was experiencing a classic case of postoperative hysteria.

"Everything's fine, Mrs. Vaughn. There's nothing wrong, believe me. It's always difficult to move the eyelids the first few days after surgery."

She calmed down, but was still anxious. "My lids," she gasped; "they hurt something terrible."

I knew that this kind of operation causes minimal pain, but to her the agony was real. It was ironic that Timmy would never see, and it didn't bother him. Mrs. Vaughn had 20/20 vision. I guess what you've never had, you never miss. I rang for the nurse and prescribed a mild pain pill, then manufactured soothing talk until she had swallowed it. Within moments, she admitted that the discomfort was gone. Still, I wrote an order on her chart requesting an ophthalmology examination before she was discharged. It would satisfy her — and it would legally cover my department.

I had deliberately planned my routine so that examination of the three new admissions, scheduled for surgery the next morning, would come last.

A face-lift, a breast augmentation (mammoplasty), and a foot ulcer. The first two were strictly cosmetic operations, I realized with considerable satisfaction. Happy surgery. Although I felt great personal fulfillment in repairing congenital defects and traumatic wounds, I had to admit there was something special about cosmetic surgery. The results were usually so dramatic, and usually the patient was so very pleased afterward.

But it was not just a matter of saving the best till last. From experience, I knew that I would have to take considerable time with each of these patients. Besides thorough histories and physicals, there would be a lot of conversation involved, and I didn't want to feel pressed.

Some surgeons tend to minimize the presurgical conference. Instead of explaining all the details and fully informing the patient of possible complications, they tell them what they have a legal right to know — but no more.

Thinking about it, I suspect there are three reasons. First, every doctor is anxious to build up his volume and is unwilling to risk scaring a patient away. Second, there's the medical mystique. Most physicians resist the idea that the patient should know or be burdened with such technicalities. The patients have placed themselves in competent hands, and that should satisfy them. Third, some surgeons simply do not want to take the time. A surgeon's financial gain is in a direct ratio to the number of patients he is able to see. While I was an intern, I had been befriended by a wealthy, elderly doctor. "Do you know the secret of running a successful private practice, son?" he'd asked. I waited, expecting words of infinite wisdom. "Never let the patient get between you and the door!" Fully explaining every operation to every patient would considerably lengthen appointment spans and result in fewer cases seen. Usually these check-and-run physicians are willing to go with the odds that a complication won't occur. And usually the odds are on their side — but they're skating on thin ice.

During my four years of general surgery residency, I

had become adept at these preliminary sessions. The most important concern was to establish and maintain an excellent rapport. I knew that a certain percentage of patients, a small percentage certainly, were going to have problems relating to their surgery. Ideally, no one should have postoperative trouble, but it doesn't work out that way. I preferred to take the most important step before the operation — informing the patient of any necessary pain or discomfort and possible complications in advance. Not only do patients have a legal right to "informed consent," but it makes sense for the doctor to anticipate human nature. If problems occur that patients have been forewarned about, they usually don't get too upset. If they have no idea that complications can occur, such developments may turn them against their doctor, plant seeds of distrust and anger — and send them hunting up the names of good malpractice attorneys.

Complete honesty is even more important in the field of cosmetic surgery than in any other specialty. Those undergoing cosmetic surgery don't *have* to have it — they *choose* to have it. If a general surgeon involved in, let's say, abdominal surgery encounters a complication or botches a procedure, he can usually correct it or, failing that, cover it up. No one except the surgical team will ever know. It is not apparent. The patient wakes up alive — his primary hope. He will probably recover and never know the difference. But complications in cosmetic surgery can cause real trouble — the patient might look worse after the operation than before. Our mistakes walk around for everyone to see.

I decided to see the augmentation mammoplasty case first. I'd just pushed open the door and stepped into the room when I nearly collided with the patient's husband, who was about to leave.

"Hi," he beamed. "I'm Bob Pearce. Tomorrow's the big day, right?" He almost danced with anticipation. "Boy-oh-boy-oh-boy! You know, doc, some fellows are leg men, but I'm a tit man myself. Make 'em big, won't you?" His hands outlined large circles in the air. "You know, like melons."

I successfully hid my distaste. How in the hell would Bob Pearce like it, I wondered, if his wife blithely announced that she was a "balls gal," a "penis freak," or an "ass woman"? Our society has established a set of unrealistic ideals, especially where women are concerned. The more a woman falls short of the ideal shown on billboards and television, the less desirable she is.

Some of our television shows are beginning to depict real people, and maybe fifty years from now Americans will feel differently. But in the meantime, I reminded myself, I'd have to deal with the world as it is. I don't make the rules of the game; I just try to make the players presentable. Nevertheless, I was glad to see Bob Pearce go.

I turned my attention to his wife, an attractive, twenty-five-year-old blonde. Her small breasts were accentuated by the fact that she was tall, almost five feet, ten inches. As I proceeded with the physical examination, her husband's comments unsettled me.

"What made you decide to have mammoplasty, Mrs. Pearce?" I asked casually.

She looked down at herself, then up at me in surprise.

"I mean, why at this particular time?"

"We just didn't have the money before." She was an extremely bright and intelligent woman, and obviously my question wasn't as subtle as I'd hoped. "Oh, are you worried that I'm doing it because of Bob?" Mrs. Pearce chuckled. "About what he said — forget it. He just likes to clown around."

She became serious. "Look, from the time I was in junior high, I had to wear a padded bra. I kept thinking that it was just a matter of maturing, that one morning I'd wake up and be the bikini type. Well, it just didn't happen. It didn't exactly ruin my life — I had lots of dates — and I didn't have any trouble snaring Bob. But don't kid yourself, doctor. In bed, no man really likes his wife to resemble a twelve-year-old."

She ran her hands lightly down her breasts. "Even being teased about them hurts. I don't have to look like Raquel Welch, but a gal needs *something* up there, just to make her clothes look right — just for her own self-esteem. The operation is for *me*." Her sincerity was evident. "Bob and I have a good marriage. He offered me this or a trip to Honolulu as a fifth anniversary present. Does that answer your question?"

"Just wanted to make sure," I admitted. "I fix bosoms — not lives."

Before I continued my examination, I withdrew from my jacket pocket a sample prosthesis, which I had brought along, and handed it to her.

"This is what we'll be using."

I watched as she took the clear, thin-walled bag containing a translucent, liquefied gel and tested its soft, fluid-like mobility. I agreed with Dr. Parmenter — it was the newest and finest prosthesis yet developed. Once implanted, it had the feel of human tissue, was almost indiscernible both to the eye and touch, and was so flexible that when a woman was lying down, it flattened slightly, just as normal breast tissue would do.

As she squeezed it and hefted it, I realized that mammoplasty had come a long way. From my studies, I knew that the first augmentation work had been done with injections of liquid silicone by needle directly into the breast. The results were often disastrous, with major and sometimes life-threatening complications. The technique is now outlawed in this country. The next method developed had utilized a Teflon sponge. But eventually that material tends to become very hard and, while medically safe, it was glaringly noticeable that an unnaturally firm and foreign substance was present. How a breast feels is as important to a woman as how it looks. Some doctors prefer to use a silicone envelope, which, once implanted, is inflated with a saline solution, but it has certain faults.

First, sometimes the valve can be felt as a hard lump. In fact, I read in a medical journal about one patient with the saline inflatable implants who had panicked her internist. He had discerned the valve during a routine physical, thought it a suspicious mass, and was readying a needle to aspirate it, a preliminary test to determine a benign or possible malignant diagnosis. Although the patient had deliberately withheld the facts up to that time, luckily she preferred that her pride be punctured rather than that part of her anatomy. Before the physician could proceed, she reluctantly admitted that her lovely breasts were not a heavenly endowment. Also, some doctors have reported that this type of prosthesis has a tendency toward leaking as time passes — a leakage as high as seven percent — not physically dangerous, but certainly "deflating." At University Hospital, the prefilled silicone gel implant was preferred.

Betty Pearce had been examining the prosthesis from all angles.

"Plastic, huh?"

"Not really. Silicone. You know," I reflected, "it's kind of unfortunate that my field is called plastic surgery, because I'd have to wrack my brain to come up with a procedure where we actually use plastic. Medically, the word *plastic* comes from the Greek *plastikos*, meaning formed or shaped."

As I'd been talking, Mrs. Pearce's sharp eyes had discerned a tiny number lightly etched on the pouch's thin covering.

"Four," she read softly, looking up. "Is that the size?"

I nodded. "They come in petite to extra large —
eight different sizes."

"Can I have my choice?"

"Within limits," I said. Unhappy experiences had
taught us that, left to their own devices, some women
would pick an outlandishly large size, having no conception of the final effect. One thing we didn't want
was an army of dissatisfied, ludicrously topheavy females as walking advertisements. "The size we implant
is worked out scientifically," I explained, "depending
on your height, weight, measurements, and the
amount of breast skin we have to work with. I'll establish a range of appropriate sizes for your build. You
can pick one of them if you like."

She thought about it. "Decisions, decisions. I'll leave
it up to you." She grinned impishly. "Gee, it's kind of
like playing God."

I chuckled and blessed her trust.

"After the operation," I advised, "we'll apply a light
dressing and a new support bra to keep the implants in
proper position. You can go home the following morning. But this is important — you are not to remove the
bra for any reason, for one week. You can use your
hands, do what you want, just don't raise your elbows
during that time. Is that clear?"

"Yes."

"After seven days, you're to come back and we'll
remove the stitches and replace the bra. For three
weeks after that, no violent movement or exercise, like

swimming or tennis, and, by the way, no sex above the waist for six weeks. Agreed?"

"Sounds reasonable. Agreed."

I took a deep breath and explained that augmentation mammoplasty is comparatively simple surgery, but complications sometimes occur. I wanted her to know about them. We discussed the possibility of hematoma, infection, and the chance of a tight capsule forming, which would give abnormal firmness. Since silicone is a foreign substance, the body always reacts by walling it off with a tissue buildup. Most of the time that tissue remains thin, and the capsule stays soft and pliable. But sometimes it becomes excessively thick. Why it happens in certain women and not in others is unknown. Perhaps some have more of a tendency to form scar tissue, or maybe they're extremely reactive to silicone. Plastic surgeons are busy researching the problem. In the meantime, it has been determined that massaging the newly implanted breast on a daily schedule has been fairly successful in preventing the formation of tight capsules. But it occurs quite often, and is the major complication.

Once I'd finished, we were both silent for several long moments.

"Is that it?" she asked.

"Can't think of anything else to scare you."

"I'm not scared. If I wanted to play it absolutely safe, I'd probably never get out of bed. Sounds to me like the odds are considerably better than venturing out on the freeway. So, as far as I'm concerned, it's full steam ahead." She hesitated. "One question. These implants — is there any possibility they can cause breast cancer?"

"Medical evidence indicates no increased incidence whatsoever."

She digested that. "We don't have any definite plans yet — but if I should have a baby . . . ?"

"Can you breast-feed it?" I anticipated her concern. "Sure. The surgery doesn't interfere with the mammary gland, it merely augments it. Function remains intact."

She relaxed with a sigh of contentment. "See you in the morning, Dr. Moynihan." I started to leave. "And, hey, don't be late!"

I nodded, grinned and left. Some patients had the ability to make your day.

My next stop was to see Mr. Nicholas Dimitrios, our sixty-seven-year-old man with a foot ulcer. Four months ago he'd had major surgery on the right hip and had recovered nicely. But weeks at home in bed had caused an open pressure sore to develop on the back of his right heel. In spite of various nonsurgical attempts to heal it, the ulcer persisted, and University Hospital's Orthopedic Department had asked us to see this patient in consultation.

A ruddy-faced man, he had dark brown and snapping eyes, and he vibrated with an air of leashed vitality.

"Mr. Dimitrios, I'm Dr. Moynihan. I'll be assisting on your surgery in the morning. Mind if I examine you and ask a few questions?" With older patients, I'd gotten into the habit of being especially deferential, rather than efficiently crisp. In our age, the elderly get little enough respect, and I'd discovered that many residents, nurses, and even senior staff physicians, who barged into a room with an "I own your body, your time, and your future welfare" attitude, were met with resentment. So why buy trouble?

"Come in, son — I mean doctor." He clicked off his television. "Glad to see you."

I gently lifted the compress bandage from his heel and saw the deep, oozing ulcer, almost an inch in diameter. Theoretically, in a hospital, bedsores are inexcusable; they denote inadequate nursing care. But it is a fact that a pressure sore can develop in an hour or two unless the patient is frequently moved and adequately padded. Good hospital personnel turn patients often and use pillows to relieve pressure points. Sheepskin coverings over sheets are employed, and water beds are becoming popular.

But Mr. Dimitrios had developed his affliction during lengthy convalescence at home. Even with a solicitous family doing their utmost, an ulcer had formed.

As I replaced the bandage, Mr. Dimitrios winced. "Sorry," I said automatically.

"Me, too," he replied. "The docs did a great job. For the first time in I don't know how many years, the hip was working fine. Then I got this damned sore heel, so I still can't walk."

"Well, we're going to take care of that," I assured

44

him. Since everything else had been tried, I explained, we had decided to repair the wound surgically with a skin flap. Step by step I outlined what he could expect. "I won't guarantee that you'll enter the Olympics," I finished, "but we'll get you back on your feet."

"We'll see." His laconic reply, in light of his cheerfulness only moments before, surprised me.

I examined him carefully, then began gathering the facts of his complicated medical history. Two heart attacks, plus a blood clot to the lung. Using general or spinal anesthesia, as we normally would for the wound procedure, presented too great a risk. Mr. Dimitrios also had a history of significant alcohol intake, and there was some evidence of senility. He was apparently a victim of mercurial moods. A note on the chart by the floor nurse indicated that only hours before, he had been expressing death wishes. He had informed her and everyone else that he wouldn't be back after surgery — he'd be going directly to the morgue. Local anesthesia for the upcoming operation was the best insurance we had that this wouldn't happen.

Outside, I picked up the chart labeled 519, and headed for the patient's room.

A rhytidectomy is the removal of wrinkles (*rhytides* in Greek), a face-lift. It was this procedure that had brought Kristina Healy to University Hospital. She was forty-six, with dark auburn hair and a body that indicated regular physical activity and exercise. She seemed a little ill at ease, as many people are once they've made the decision in favor of cosmetic surgery.

45

Soul-searching is inevitable while the patient strives to justify the extravagance of spending considerable money on what could be called sheer vanity and self-indulgence. Coupled with that indecision is the fact that, for perhaps the very first time in her life, a woman is forced to admit to herself that she is middle-aged. After all, no truly young woman needs a face-lift — and to some, it's a depressing, bitter realization.

I completed the history and physical, then asked the routine psychological question.

"What made you decide on a face-lift, Mrs. Healy?"

"I had lunch with my mother," she said cryptically, in a flat tone. My upraised eyebrows forced her to continue.

"Mom was twenty when I was born, and the whole time I was growing up, everyone remarked on how much we resembled each other. She lives in the East now, but she was flying to Hawaii last month and stopped over in Los Angeles for a couple of days." Mrs. Healy was silent for a few moments as she reflected. "Mother told me how well I looked. I'm afraid I couldn't return the compliment. I guess we talked about everything under the sun, but it was all kind of a blur. I only remember staring at her wrinkles. Directly opposite me was an image of myself a few years from now. I actually rushed home and headed straight for a mirror. It was like a bad dream come true. Jowls! I had jowls! And lines, I counted every one of them. And the skin around my eyes — I was starting to look like a boozer." The confession hurt and she found it easy to change the subject.

"My husband was killed nine years ago, and there's nobody to support me but myself. I'm talent coordinator on one of the TV talk shows. It's a fast-paced, interesting, good-paying job — and I intend to keep it."

"Fair enough," I said.

"Is it?" Her teeth caught her lower lip. "I've had some doubts. You know what finally convinced me? My daughter's eighteen, and she's the only one I've told about this. Poor kid, I've nearly driven her up the wall. First I'd announce I was going through with the face-lift routine; the next minute, I'd change my mind. Finally she just about blew her top. She reminded me how strict I'd been about her wearing braces on her teeth when she was a kid. And she wanted to know what was so different about spending money to improve the looks of her teeth — or having surgery to improve the appearance of my face. So I thought about it, and she was right. Anyway, here I am."

Well, Mrs. Healy had passed my little test with flying colors, and I wanted to ease any doubts she might still be harboring.

"Face-lifts work, Mrs. Healy. Often a person looks ten or fifteen years younger. I think you'll be happy with the results."

I went on to explain that her rhytidectomy would be done with heavy sedation and a local anesthetic, and began outlining each step. From the questions she asked, I realized she had considerable knowledge about the planned procedure. Apparently her job required meticulous research, and she had applied the same

47

technique in ferreting out facts about face-lifts. Nothing I told her came as any great surprise.

"Of course, for a few weeks, you'll look like you just went four rounds with the middleweight champion — but the bruises and swelling will gradually disappear."

"I know. No problem. The show is on a six-week hiatus, so that'll work out fine."

"And no chewing for two or three days. Liquids only. Avoid any activity that might stretch the facial skin or muscles and pull the stitches loose. It's a good idea to sleep on your back."

She nodded. "So I've heard."

"Are you aware of the possible complications involved?" I asked.

For the first time her eyes became troubled. "The articles I've read, and the people I've talked to, they didn't mention any. . . ."

It was typical for tabloid and magazine features to extol the advantages of face-lifts and to ignore the discomforts and risks. I guess authors have discovered that upbeat articles sell better.

However, I had a responsibility, so I reviewed with her the possible complications such as bleeding and infection.

"If that's the worst that can happen . . . ," she said thoughtfully.

"It isn't. There's more. There are five branches of the facial nerve. The biggest danger is an injury to the one that controls the forehead muscles. If that happens, it results in the inability to wrinkle the forehead on one side."

She had a nice laugh. "Well, in my business, not being able to frown might be an asset. Seriously, what do you do if that happens?"

"Usually, in time, function returns. If it doesn't, we have two options. Theoretically, we can reoperate and stitch the cut ends of the nerve branch back together. It's a very difficult procedure and results are usually unsatisfactory. The most practical solution is to go in and cut the same branch on the other side so the forehead can't wrinkle at all. At least that way it's symmetrical."

The complication I had described occurred rarely, but as I'd been talking to Mrs. Healy I'd remembered hearing of a similar incident at another hospital. As usual in teaching hospitals, the staff plastic surgeon had done one side of a face while a resident was doing the other, and, since the patient had been under local anesthetic, she had been dimly aware of the dual technique. As luck would have it, it had been the staff surgeon who had inadvertently cut through the temporal branch during the procedure. Such an injury is usually not discovered during the operation; it becomes apparent only as the face heals. Anyway, the patient, once aware of the unfortunate results, had ranted and raved. Damn that resident, she had stormed. It was gross incompetence! He hadn't known what he was doing! The side of the forehead *he* had done still had wrinkles when she frowned. She insisted on the same lovely unlined effect on both sides! Unwilling to admit his error, the surgeon had quickly agreed, cut the temporal nerve on the other side, and sent the patient home extolling his virtues — but still cursing the amateurish ineptness of the hapless resident.

I glanced up and saw an expression of fleeting concern. "There's still time," I reminded Mrs. Healy gently. "Do you want to think about it?"

"No. I just hope it's worth it."

I swung the service table across her bed and propped up a hand mirror so she could see her reflection. Then, leaning across behind her, I spread my fingers in front of her ears and along the temples, pulling back and up on her facial skin and tissue. The change was remarkable. She suddenly looked at least ten years younger.

"That's just to give you the general effect," I said.

"How long will it last?" she whispered.

"It varies. Maybe eight to ten years. Face-lifts remove the traces of previous years, but they can't retard future aging. We can turn back the clock, but we can't stop it."

I started to leave. "See you tomorrow." When I didn't get a reply, I glanced back. Mrs. Healy had placed her fingers where mine had been and was exerting the same kind of pressure. The anticipatory smile on her face was the sort of thing that made my profession worthwhile.

Chapter Three

I T WAS AFTER FIVE before I'd finished, so I headed for the doctors' lounge. At this hour, I knew I wouldn't be alone. It didn't take long for the house staff physicians to learn that dodging food carts and competing with dinner trays was a waste of time. The lounge was also popular during visiting hours, for making rounds then was the sign of a true novice. The hapless resident would be peppered with questions from the patient's family and friends, squandering interminable time on meaningless dialogue. During these periods, there was a constantly changing group in the lounge. After resting for five or ten minutes, some of the doctors would be lured away by the page or urgent duties, and their places were quickly taken by others. The banter and discussions, while almost always shop talk, were invariably stimulating and amusing.

A few of the single residents lived at the hospital. I

didn't. During my third year at medical school in St. Louis I'd gone to a fraternity party and spied a blond girl who stood out from the rest. I introduced myself and struck up a conversation. I discovered that Patsy Saunders had attended Barat College, a women's school at Lake Forest, Illinois, but had recently transferred to the local university for a year. I got the number of her college dorm and a few days later called her for a date. She accepted. I figured maybe my blue eyes and dark hair had turned the trick. Much later, Patsy admitted that she hadn't been wearing her glasses that night — she had no idea what I looked like. But whatever attracted her to me, I knew what attracted me to her. Sweetness, sophistication, and gentility. *Everyone* seemed to like Patsy, and *I* liked that. Plus, thank God, she had nothing to do with medicine; she added balance to my life. At the time, they were good reasons, but I know now I would have married her no matter what. I loved her! But during that period, I was determined to stay single until I was thirty and a trained surgeon. Patsy decided to return to Illinois and got her bachelor's degree in English literature, and then went on to Manhattanville College for her master's in teaching, with a specialization in Montessori education. For four years after we met, we wrote and called each other occasionally, and I halfheartedly played the field. But while I was serving my first year of general surgery residency and Patsy was teaching at a school in Cambridge, Massachusetts, she was able to vacation in California. Two days after she arrived, I decided to throw in the bachelor's towel. We were married in the fall of my second year at University Hospital.

I still chuckle when I recall our wedding, for it was so typical of Patsy's velvet-gloved determination. Her all-time favorite film is *Love Story,* and she had made up her mind that we would be married in the Memorial Church, like Ryan O'Neal and Ali McGraw. When I pointed out that it was impossible, that only Harvard students were permitted to use that facility, she promptly enrolled in some obscure extension class Harvard was offering — "The Culture and Civilization of Nigeria," I think — and paid her seventeen-dollar-and-fifty-cents registration fee. Then, receipt in hand, she trotted across the Harvard Yard and promptly booked the chapel for our wedding.

On our return to California, we were lucky enough to find an apartment within the required ten minutes' driving distance from the medical center and had settled into a comfortable routine. Medicine is a jealous mistress, and I was determined that although it might have most of my time, it wouldn't get all of it.

I usually arrived at the hospital between five-thirty and six A.M. Rounds were made in the morning and late afternoon. Every patient on our service was seen twice a day. Conversation to determine any medical complaints, removing stitches, changing bandages, and writing new orders take time — and it wasn't unusual to have twenty patients hospitalized by our department on any given day. Of course, Parmenter and

Burke and I shared these duties, for it was important that we all have contact with every patient so they'd feel at ease with any one of us. Nevertheless, as resident, I drew the major responsibility for rounds. Every other night I was on call. This didn't mean that I was required to stay on the hospital premises, but it did mean that I must be readily available to answer questions, change orders or return to the hospital for emergencies. I wore a "beeper," a paging device that had a radius of about twenty miles, so I could be contacted. I soon learned that I could expect about ten night calls a week — not a great volume, but the trouble was that I never knew *when* they'd come or what the emergency might be.

I remember one night Patsy and I had dinner reservations at a favorite French restaurant, and just as we were walking out our door I got a call. Parmenter had performed an otoplasty that morning on an outpatient — an operation that corrected protruding ears. Once he got home, the patient's left ear had begun oozing blood, and I said that I would meet him at the Emergency Room immediately. Since Patsy was all dressed, and it might save us time, she went with me. She sat in the E.R. waiting room, surrounded by the mauled and maimed, while I reanesthetized the incision in the patient's ear, took the stitches out, cauterized the bleeders, and closed. It took over an hour. We had just reached the restaurant's parking lot when I got another call. The patient's other ear was oozing. I couldn't believe it. I had inspected the right ear as well, and it had looked fine. But back we went to the hospital, where I spent an additional hour on the other ear. By the time I'd finished, it was well after eleven o'clock — and Patsy and I congratulated each other on being lucky enough to find a pizza joint open.

After that, I just didn't plan anything for the nights I was on call. It was easier that way.

Besides rounds and being on call, I helped man the plastic surgery clinic on Tuesdays and Thursdays. We operated Mondays, Wednesdays, and Fridays. In between, I managed to take histories and physicals on newly admitted patients. While I supposedly had every other weekend off, I still made morning rounds on those Saturdays and Sundays, and caught up on any paperwork left undone.

During the week, even though it made for a long day, I almost always stuck around until seven P.M., just in case there were any last-minute problems.

Today was no different, so I took a battered-looking jelly doughnut, drew a cup of coffee from the urn, and joined the group in the lounge. The others looked up, nodded their welcome, but didn't interrupt an intern named Rafe Lamotta, who was in the middle of a story.

". . . As medical students go, I'd say Reardon is really gung-ho." The others nodded and he went on. "Anyway, he's been bugging the O.B. resident to let him sew up an episiotomy. This birth had been strictly routine and Greg decided to give him his chance — told him to go ahead. When I came into the delivery room, there was Reardon, bent over, concentrating like mad.

He was anxious to do everything just right, and his face was just a few inches from the patient's vulva. He was doing okay, but as he swung the needle around, he looped the catgut through one of his mask ties. He didn't know it and went right on sewing. When he finished and tried to straighten up, he discovered his mask was sutured to the woman's vulva. That was one surprised kid."

We all roared with laughter.

"What happened?" asked Bob Bruckman, one of the physical therapists.

"Nurse Boswick to the rescue. She cut him loose."

Dr. Buckley Phillips, a psychiatry intern, entered the room and flopped into a chair. Psychiatrists were a breed apart, I'd discovered. While most of the interns and residents on the other services were conservative, with closely cropped hair, white lab coats, and subdued ties, psychiatric residents went to the other extreme. They were sort of the hippies of the medical profession. Dr. Phillips was no exception. His loud sport shirt was adorned with love beads and a medallion, and his hair curled almost to his shoulders.

"Hi, Buck," I said.

He scowled. "No pleasantries, please. Especially not from surgeons."

"What's bugging *you*?" someone asked.

"I just told you — *surgeons*." He sighed. "I just got a call from the fourth floor. They've got a gallbladder patient who's kind of flipped out. They called me to consult. You know what that yo-yo who passes himself off as the surgical resident told me? 'Come down and fix it,' he says. Fix it! Like I could just cut out the guy's psychiatric problem like — like an appendix, or something."

I smiled. Any university hospital is more a collection of different departments than a unified facility. It manages to function, but the loyalty of each member of a specialty is directed to his own department rather than the hospital as a whole. Competition is real, and a kind of tongue-in-cheek antagonism is always present. For instance, surgeons refer to Internal Medicine residents as "the herbs and roots boys." We imply that they've risen just one step above witchcraft with their potions and treatments. They retaliate by saying that our motto is "If it can't be cut, it can't be cured!" Even Psychiatry's electrotherapy treatment center wasn't immune. At our hospital, it was known as the Thomas Edison Memorial Wing. Radiologists were "rads," pediatricians were referred to as "pedipods," and the urologists were called "plumbers."

Before Buck could continue complaining, Dr. Moser, an intern from Orthopedics, poked his head through the door.

"Hey! Has anybody seen Dr. Dedrick?"

Boyd Falmouth, the senior resident from the General Surgery Department, raised his head.

"Come off it, Junior. You know it's after five. Dedrick's half way to the country club by now."

"Oh. Yeah. Sorry." Dr. Moser shrugged and backed out of the room.

57

Falmouth felt our eyes on him. "Dedrick and his nine-to-five brand of medicine drives me up the wall," he said. "As far as I'm concerned, being a doctor means twenty-four-hour-a-day responsibility. Dedrick missed his calling. He should have been an auto mechanic or a steel worker."

I shifted to look at him. "Let's face it, there are doctors and there are doctors. Let me tell you a story. You're not going to believe this, but it's absolutely true. It happened while I was in medical school in St. Louis. There was this cancer surgeon — Dr. Langdon. He was very good. Very finicky and compulsive — and very slow. I was assisting in operating room A with a duodenal ulcer. Langdon was in room B with a kidney carcinoma. Both cases had an eight A.M. start. We finished about eleven. Langdon was still working. Next morning I arrived around seven A.M. to scrub in, and noticed Langdon was operating in room B. 'Boy, he got an early start,' I said to the surgical supervisor. She shook her head." I glanced around the room and noticed I had everyone's full attention. "Would you believe Langdon was still doing the same kidney patient? When he got in, he found the malignancy had spread. He removed a kidney and a lobe of the liver — and chased that damned cancer all the way up into the diaphragm. Then he had to repair. A twenty-three-hour operation! It had to be a record."

"Boy!" breathed Dr. Phillips.

"So," I finished, "there are the Dedricks and then there are the Langdons, right?"

"What about the patient?" Boyd asked. "Did he live?"

"You bet he lived."

Young Stephen Vance, just a year away from graduating and beginning his internship, hovered at the door. Since it was a teaching institution, our hospital teemed with medical students. After being accepted by the affiliated school, they spent the first two years in classes. Then, possessing the fundamental knowledge, they were exposed to clinical situations within the hospital — to listen, to learn, to observe, and to do — all under strict supervision. Aware of his status as a student, Steve stood diffidently. He was unwilling to intrude and was unsure of his welcome — but he was hoping to be invited to join the big kids.

"Did you hear about the big flap up on seven?" he asked.

We hadn't, and were always hungry for gossip. Protocol and pecking order be damned. We waved him in.

"What's happening?" Rafe demanded.

"Some Demerol's missing from the cardiac unit," Steve whispered. "A lot of it. The way they figure, one of the doctors must be an addict. You never saw such a commotion." We were uncomfortably silent, and Steve went on. "I don't understand it. A doctor! Knowing what he knows — how could he let himself get hooked?"

"Pressure," Boyd said quietly.

"Availability," I added.

59

Steve shook his head. "But it's so dumb. Once you have that degree, you've got it made. Everything else just falls in place —"

Rafe had been thumbing through the latest issue of *JAMA,* the monthly *Journal of the American Medical Association.* The last few pages always listed the physician members who had died that month. Each had a brief obituary, which included the cause of death. Rafe found the section and shoved it toward Steve.

"Take a look," he commanded. "Sure, there are heart attacks and accidents and all the rest. But take a good look." He pointed. "See here — and here — and here? A lot of barbiturate overdoses and self-inflicted gunshot wounds. Right?"

Steve peered at the pages with widening eyes. "I don't get it."

"They had it made," Rafe said. "You work and work, and you get where you want to be — and then you discover the price is too high."

Any further discussion was cut off by the blast of the paging system.

"Dr. Moynihan, please. Dr. Donald Moynihan."

I reached for the phone, identified myself, and was told that I was needed in the Emergency Room. With a quick good-bye salute to the others, I trotted out the door.

As I have said, life in a teaching hospital is partly a series of political maneuvers. For a surgeon to be well trained in his field, he must be exposed to many and varied patients, and as the plastic surgery resident competing with all the other services, I knew I'd have to fight for my cases and personally make sure that a sufficient variety came my way.

Toward that end, I'd made periodic visits to the Emergency Room, becoming friendly with the doctors and nurses working there, even cheerfully helping out when they were shorthanded. I'd mentioned the kind of patients that interested me, and I'd assured them I'd be happy to come to the E.R. any time, regardless of the hour or circumstances. They were pleasantly surprised, and they'd promised to keep me in mind. If I was called and saw the patient first, the case was mine. In this game, what you see is what you get.

Entering the E.R., I sensed that the receptionist was a bit ruffled, but was striving to maintain her composure and dignity. Her voice was tight.

"Examining room number four, Dr. Moynihan," she directed.

I walked across and was forced to pause at the entrance. The small area was teeming with people — the Emergency Room doctor, three nurses, a team of X-ray technicians with portable equipment, an orderly, two policemen, and two sailors. Somewhere behind that mass was the patient. I had to wedge and elbow my way through.

As soon as he saw me, the Emergency Room doctor smiled. "He's all yours. I've got three other cases waiting. It's a busy night." And he disappeared.

The odor of stale beer nearly knocked me over. Lying on the gurney was another sailor. His face was a mess, but a wide grin shone through the encrusted blood. It was obvious that he was feeling no pain. As I started my examination, I could feel the crowd in the small room pressing in on me.

"All right," I said, "everybody but the nurses and orderly will have to wait outside," and I pulled the curtains to screen off the room. The nurses helped clean the wounds with soap and sterile water, and draped the area around the patient's face.

My probing revealed multiple lacerations of his lips and forehead. Most of the cuts were superficial, but several were fairly deep. I was also sure he had a broken cheekbone, which the X-rays would confirm. But the first order of business was getting his lacerations sewed — and I sighed at the prospect. I'd had experiences with drunks before, and they could be taxing. The correct amount of sedation to give someone utterly inebriated is difficult to determine. Better that I order none than to have him develop breathing problems.

I settled for injecting small amounts of Novocain, and while I waited for it to take effect, I learned that the victim's name was Wayne Banker. Just that day he'd been promoted to the rank of Chief Petty Officer and he and his two friends, also chiefs, had wangled three-day passes from the nearby naval base. They'd decided to celebrate in a rough area of town called the Combat Zone and had proceeded to get roaring drunk in a sleazy bar. Wayne had moved in on somebody's girl, a heated argument had erupted, and the bartender had slammed a baton, which he kept handy for scuffles, across Banker's face.

I had just started suturing when one of the sailors pushed back the curtain and stepped just inside.

"How's he doing, doc?"

Wayne suddenly sat bolt upright on the table. Naturally, the drapes, sheets, and towels that insured sterility flew in every direction.

"Barney," he shouted to his pal, "let's go back and get that son-of-a-bitch!" I pushed him firmly back on the table. The nurse got fresh draping.

"Naw," Barney replied. I glanced up in time to see him lean against the wall and, as if in slow motion, gently slide down it until he was sitting on the floor. I noticed an ugly bruise on his neck in the vicinity of his Adam's apple, and another high on one cheek. I gestured to one of the hovering nurses to attend him.

"How did you get the bruises, Barney?" I asked, all the while carefully stitching Wayne's face.

"The fuckin' cop!" Barney exploded. "He did it! I didn't do nothing, and he worked me over in the squad car!!"

"Take him, Barney, take him," Wayne Banker yelled, struggling to rise. I pushed him back.

A policeman charged into the room. "He's lying! I never laid a hand on him!"

I hastily handed the needle holder to the nurse and rushed between Barney and the cop. The hell with sterility. With so many people milling about, it was ridiculous to bother.

"Peggy!" I called to one of the nurses. "Get an ice pack for Barney's neck and stick with him." I waited until she hurried over. "And when you get a chance," I whispered, "have somebody call the Shore Patrol. He'll probably be safer with them than with that goon." Then I whirled and glared at the officer until he resumed his position just outside the door.

I took a couple more stitches as Peggy knelt to apply the cold compress. As she did, the sailor obviously grabbed a handful of her anatomy, because she shrieked.

"Dammit, behave yourself, Barney!" I ordered. I'd just resumed suturing Wayne again when, out of the corner of my eye, I saw Barney grab at the nylon-sheathed ankle of a passing nurse. The exertion caused him to throw up, spewing the evening's beer over the nurse and in all directions. I tersely suggested that the orderly get a kidney basin and replace Peggy.

"Let's hope you're not his type," I said.

The other police officer, while more rational than his partner, seemed obsessed with getting a signature — any signature — on his report. Time after time he wandered in, approaching me, the nurses, and even the orderly, with papers extended, his eyes pleading.

"Will you please wait outside and just stay out of the way?" I suggested.

As the curtains parted, I saw the third sailor, sitting quietly in the hall on a chair. I looked at him and noticed huge tears streaming down his face.

"What's your name, sailor?" I called.

"Robert. Robert Halpern," he sobbed.

"Are you hurt?"

He shook his head, spattering tears in all directions.

"Then what's the matter? Your buddies are going to be okay."

"They'll bust us," he wailed. "We'll lose our rank."

"While you're waiting, doc, could you just sign this?" The compulsive police officer had entered and was resuming his crusade. My patience suddenly ran out.

"The next person who comes into this room or opens his mouth is going to find himself flat on his ass," I roared.

The nurses and orderly stared at me, properly shocked, but I had found a language that the sailors and policemen understood. Even when the Shore Patrol arrived, they stood outside, talking in whispers.

It had taken over two and a half hours. The X-rays confirmed a broken cheekbone. I had Wayne admitted. We would either operate to reduce the fracture in a few days, or Chief Banker would be transferred to a military hospital for the procedure.

By the time I had cleaned up, charted orders and double-checked on my patient, it was past ten-thirty. I reached for the phone and dialed my home number.

"Patsy? Hi. Sorry I couldn't call before. Got tied up with an emergency."

"That's okay," she said cheerily.

"What's for dinner?"

"Well — I *had* a pot roast —"

"I'll just grab a cheeseburger on my way home."

I chose an all-night diner at random, and as I waited I realized that I was falling prey to the plastic surgeon's occupational disease — seeing prospective patients everywhere I looked. The fry cook had a prominent jutting jaw, a congenital malformation of the mandible. The young man who served me, besides having acne, also suffered from a poorly repaired harelip. After a few bites of the sandwich, my appetite evaporated.

It was time to go home.

Chapter Four

I ARRIVED AT THE HOSPITAL before six the next morning so that I could make rounds before the scheduled surgery. Wayne Banker was snoring away the effects of the evening before, Betty Pearce had been properly sedated for her upcoming operation, and all the other patients were on an even keel. I headed for the Surgical Supervisor's station on the ninth floor and studied the procedures board where our three patients were listed. Mrs. Pearce's augmentation mammoplasty was scheduled for eight A.M., Mrs. Healy's face-lift was set to go at ten, and the repair of Mr. Dimitrios's heel ulcer was indicated for three P.M. Opposite each procedure, in the column headed "Surgeon," was the notation: "Parmenter/Burke/Moynihan," but I knew that the two staff men conferred each evening and discussed the division of cases. As I was checking the O.R. assignments, the Chief of Plastic Surgery came up behind me.

"You'll be assisting me on the breasts and the face-lift," Dr. Parmenter said casually, "then you can help our number two man with the heel flap."

I grinned. I could imagine Burke's chagrin at being thrown the reconstructive procedure rather than a chance to perfect his technique on the cosmetic cases that would be his bread and butter once he got into private practice. But rank has its privileges.

"You go ahead," Parmenter suggested. "I have to phone my stockbroker."

As soon as I had scrubbed, I entered the O.R. Mrs. Pearce was lying on the table. She was prepped and draped, leaving only the operating field exposed. The circulating nurse, holding the gown, waited until I had strapped on my "headlight."

Not all plastic surgeons use this device, but I had learned of its value from an ear, nose, and throat man with whom I had previously worked. It was a high-intensity lamp, about an inch in diameter, held in place by a strap around my head. It had been designed with a ball-bearing joint, and I took a moment to focus and test the concentrated beam. Naturally, every operating room is equipped with adjustable overhead lights, and it is the circulating nurse's job to be sure that they are always in a position for maximum illumination of the operative field. But although they are strong and powerful, their actual size diffuses the light, and sometimes the circulator becomes distracted by other urgent duties. However, by a slight movement of my head, I could direct my headlight at a particular angle and have intensified illumination exactly where I wanted it.

So, with the headlight adjusted, gowned, gloved, and my mask in place, I approached Mrs. Pearce. She was in a heavy sedation-induced sleep, her breathing deep and regular.

"A number twenty-six needle, please," I requested, and began injecting into the breast a mixture of Xylocaine, a local anesthetic, and epinephrine, a drug that reduces bleeding by constricting the blood vessels.

Xylocaine is effective within two or three minutes, but it takes approximately eight minutes for epinephrine to work. Parmenter timed it almost perfectly. When he entered, Mrs. Pearce's right breast was already blanched white.

The Chief of Plastic Surgery glanced at my headlight and grinned. While he admitted its value, he personally found one encumbering and a nuisance.

"Ready to go, coal miner?" he joked. I smiled in return and nodded.

Dr. Parmenter took a blue marking pen and carefully outlined the proposed incisions at the edge of the dark area under the lower half of each nipple. Once he had made the small semicircular slit in the right breast, I placed the retractors to stretch the opening and make access easier, then began cauterizing the bleeders. General surgeons usually use a pencil-shaped electrocautery, but we used a forceps-like instrument that simultaneously pinched the blood vessel and supplied the necessary heat for coagulation. Parmenter carefully began dissecting between the back of the mammary gland and the chest wall muscle to create the pocket that would house the implant.

There was very little conversation during the procedure. Some surgeons, with their patients under general anesthesia, indulge in casual conversation, off-color jokes, and hospital gossip. But with a patient under local anesthesia, even though he or she apparently is asleep, there is no way of judging what might be picked up subliminally. Therefore, we even studiously avoided mentioning upsetting words like *blood* or *cut*.

The prostheses had been removed from their packages, the nurse had placed them on towels in an open tray and subjected them to our "flash" autoclave for three minutes at 270 degrees Fahrenheit. Now the implants were immersed in a basin containing saline solution.

Parmenter meticulously ascertained that there was no bleeding. Then, taking one of the prosthetic devices, he began inserting it. The incision was small, and I marveled as he expertly kneaded and maneuvered the implant, slowly, a little at a time, until it was properly seated, finally slipping his fingers between it and the breast tissue to make sure it was symmetrical and aligned with the nipple. He closed the skin with what we call "buried" stitches, which run the length of the incision, just underneath the skin. This avoids cross-hatching or a railroad-tie effect. Since the incision was made at the juncture of the areola, the dark area around the nipple, it would heal more quickly than one in the breast fold. Except for a slight redness, the scar would be almost undetectable in about eight weeks.

Dr. Parmenter straightened for a moment as I cleansed the incision with hydrogen peroxide, then placed Vaseline-impregnated gauze over it.

"Mrs. Pearce?" Dr. Parmenter called. When there was no response, he glanced at me. "Why don't you do the other breast, Don?"

While he watched closely, occasionally making a suggestion, assisting me as I had assisted him, I duplicated the procedure. It took me slightly longer, but I was pleased that my workmanship equaled his. In the months to come, I would do many, many, augmentation mammoplasties, but my success on this particular morning would remain vivid.

Now that the surgery was finished, Steri-strips were taped across the incision and a light gauze dressing was applied. Mrs. Pearce would be fitted with a supportive bra and sent to the Recovery Room until she awakened.

And she would awaken with a greatly improved silhouette. What nature had been unable to provide in twenty-five years, we had managed to accomplish in an hour and a half.

We had time to spare before the next operation, and Dr. Parmenter and I headed to the lounge for coffee. We'd been seated for only a few minutes when Dr. Roger Longstreet appeared. Longstreet was a locally prominent psychiatrist who was occasionally called in to consult at University Hospital.

"Larry," he said enthusiastically as he pumped Parmenter's hand, "long time no see. I heard about your surgical triumph last month. That was quite a feat. So what have you done recently to top it?"

Parmenter gazed at him blandly. "Triumph? What triumph do you mean? There are so many, you know."

Longstreet went along with the game. "If you have any faults, Larry, I'd have to say they're modesty and humbleness. You know the one — that reconstruction of the esophagus you did. I understand you used some penis skin for the graft."

"Uh huh."

"Any complications?" Longstreet pressed.

"Not really," Parmenter drawled. "It went just fine. The only problem is that every time my patient sees a good-looking chick, he gets a stiff neck."

I joined in the laughter. The Chief of Plastic Surgery was kidding, but I actually knew of a young woman who'd suffered a severe burn on her lip. The disfiguring wound was reconstructed by using a mucosal graft from the lining of her vagina. It's an acceptable procedure for repair, since the textures closely match, and the result was quite satisfying. There was only one slightly embarrassing complication. The color of her lip changed to a purplish hue every twenty-eight days, during her menstrual period.

I used the few minutes before scrubbing to examine the medical photographs attached to Kristina Healy's records. There were full-face shots, profiles, and three-quarter views, showing her face in repose and in animation. I studied them carefully, knowing they would be helpful in deciding the amount of undermining that should be done.

By the time Dr. Parmenter and I were ready to be gowned and gloved, Mrs. Healy was already in the O.R., sound asleep. This particular room, instead of having the usual surgical table, had been modified and the patient was resting in a sort of dental chair, her arms and legs gently restrained to prevent involuntary movement. This semisitting position, with the head and shoulders raised at perhaps a thirty-degree angle, decreases bleeding. The loose skin folds also show up better.

I shaved a strip just above Mrs. Healy's ear and well behind the hairline, careful to limit the area to the amount of skin to be excised. That way, the final suture lines would be undetectable. I drew the hair upward into a ponytail, secured it with rubber bands, and stitched a sterile towel over it. A thick application of antibacterial ointment to the exposed hairline insured that no loose strands would fall into our field of operation.

Dr. Parmenter, using the blue marking pen, expertly designed the planned incision, tracing a line downward along the shaved area, extending it in front of the ear in the natural fold, the preauricular crease, curving it under the earlobe and up directly behind the ear, finally sloping it into the hair at the nape of the neck. Then I proceeded with the anesthetizing injections while Parmenter studied the photographs.

After waiting for the Xylocaine to take effect, Dr.

73

Parmenter used a scalpel to cut along the premarked blueprint. Then, working downward from each incision line, he began undermining.

Undermining is the key to the effectiveness of a face-lift. The surgeon makes a large facial flap by cutting through the fat just under the skin, completely freeing it from the underlying tissue. It can be done with surgical scissors, a scalpel, or "bluntly" with fingers wrapped in a gauze pad to provide tension. The skin is totally loosened from the temple to the outer end of the eyebrow, over the cheeks, and halfway down the neck. Then, the skin flap is laid back to expose the underlying tissue. Any laxness in the muscle tissue is made more firm by a number of strategically placed stitches in the fascia, and temporarily laid the loose lying over the muscles of the face and neck. The skin flap is then pulled up and back. It is easy to see that the more area undermined, the greater the improvement.

Parmenter undermined the right side, placed the stitches in the fascia, and temporarily laid the loose flap of skin back into its original position. He turned Mrs. Healy's head to allow access to the other side and nodded at me to duplicate the procedure. When my undermining and stitches exactly matched his own, Parmenter went back to the original side, pulled the skin up and back, and marked the excess, which would be trimmed away. Removing exactly the proper amount of skin is important to this procedure. If too little is trimmed away, some facial sagging will remain. If too much is removed, there is too much tension, which results in an undesirable, "tight" facial appearance. Once he had finished, I repeated the process on what I now termed "my side." It had taken Parmenter an hour and a half. I had duplicated the procedure in just under two hours. With the surgery completed, Dr. Parmenter took a few steps back to survey the overall effect.

"Nice, very nice."

I wasn't sure whether the Chief of Plastic Surgery was referring to his handiwork or mine. I would later realize that he demanded and expected perfection. Words of praise seldom passed his lips, but anything short of his expectations provoked a tantrum not soon to be forgotten.

"Would you apply the dressing?" he said.

I began winding lengths of gauze around my hand, forming doughnut-shaped pads, which would protect each of the patient's ears. Gauze fluffs were made in order to apply pressure, which would insure quick adhesion of the skin to the underlying tissue. Then I wound layers of gauze roll and Ace bandages around the patient's face and neck, securing them with copious amounts of tape. When I'd finished, Mrs. Healy was swathed in a substantial dressing that looked like a football helmet.

I managed to get to the cafeteria a little before two and had almost finished my lunch when Dr. Lou Augustine, a third-year resident in Internal Medicine, joined me at the table. Lou was tall, muscular, black, and a very complex individual. He often adopted a wryly irreverent and cynical attitude, but it was actually a facade that covered a dedicated and extremely talented physician. I'd caught him cradling an injured child and seen tears rolling down his cheeks, yet in the next breath he was cracking a joke to hide his deep feelings. Not too many people knew that Lou's brother was a world-famous basketball star, or that his sister was one of the city's three black municipal judges. As he sat down I was surprised that, for once, Lou seemed utterly serious and a little excited.

"Hey," he blurted, "did you hear the news? They've just discovered the cause of sickle-cell anemia!" This is a genetic blood disease that has baffled doctors through the ages — a serious, debilitating illness that is only found among members of the black race.

"Jesus," I breathed. "That's great. What's the cause?"

"The glue on the back of food stamps!" His burst of laughter filled the room, causing heads all over the cafeteria to turn in our direction. I grinned and shook my head.

"Very funny," I said. "Have me paged when you need another straight man."

As I left the room, I saw Lou pick up his tray and join an intern at another table — who I'm sure he hoped was as gullible as I had been.

I stopped at Admitting and was told that our service's only new patient had already checked in. If I hurried, I could do a partial workup on him before the heel flap surgery scheduled for three.

SKIN DEEP: THE MAKING OF A PLASTIC SURGEON

The carbon copy of the admitting slip that I'd
picked up supplied minimal information. Anthony
Rocco — room 619 — facial scar revision — primary
surgeon, Dr. Lawrence Parmenter. I asked the floor
nurse for the patient's records and was handed a chart
almost two inches thick. Suddenly the name rang a
bell. Tony Rocco. I'd seen this patient briefly while
doing the plastic surgery rotation during my general
surgery residency, and I spent a few minutes skimming
his chart to reestablish the case in my mind.

Three days after graduating from college, Tony had
joined the police academy and had breezed through
the rigorous training. He'd been on the streets for
about a year when he and his partner answered the
silent alarm at a motel. Once on the scene, the two
officers had crouched behind the protection of their
opened car doors, guarding the only exit, and waited
for backup units. But the thief inside had come out
firing, and the shotgun blast had ricocheted, knocking
off half of Patrolman Rocco's lower jaw, part of his
tongue, and a large area of his throat. He had been in
the hospital many, many times for multiple operations.

The jaw had been reconstructed through a series of
bone grafts and skin flaps, and a tracheostomy — a tube
implanted in the windpipe, which enabled him to
breathe through his neck rather than his mouth and
nose — had been performed. Unfortunately, repairing
his tongue was beyond our craft. The part that remained was insufficient to push food back against his
palate and into his throat. In other words, Tony was

77

unable to swallow. The surgeons had done the best they could. A gastrostomy had followed, with a tube placed directly through the abdominal wall into Tony's stomach so that he could feed himself, but the food had to be limited to bottles of specially formulated liquid.

Armed with the information, I entered the room and was greeted with a wide grin by the young dark-haired man lying in bed. Although the skin over his jaw was scarred, his appearance was fairly acceptable. A pert woman sat in the chair nearby.

"Hi, I'm Dr. Moynihan."

"Sure, I remember you." Before Tony spoke, his hand had automatically risen to his throat, and his fingers covered the trach tube, cutting off the air exit, allowing him to speak. Even so, the words were slurred and slow. "This is my wife, Vicky."

I moved around the bed to shake hands with Mrs. Rocco, then turned back to the patient.

"How are you doing?" I asked.

"Pretty good." The fingertips of his other hand lightly caressed an ugly facial scar, an unavoidable holdover from previous surgery. "Took vacation, came in to have this fixed."

"Bring me up to date," I said. "It's been a long time."

"Two years," he croaked. "Two years since the shooting."

Tony's wife wet her lips and entered the conversation, obviously anxious to spare her husband the agony

78

of telling a long story. She managed to help out as her husband's voice so tactfully that it was not emasculating.

"Tony got a medical retirement from the police force," she began, "and the pension wasn't bad. I told him if we were careful we could get along on it, but..."

"Get along, hell," Tony interrupted. "I'm only twenty-four. I owe more than just 'getting along' to my wife and kid...."

"Anyway," Vicky continued, "Tony finally landed a spot as a part-time estimator with the real estate department of a local bank. It pays pretty well."

"That's great," I said enthusiastically.

Tony propped himself up on one elbow and made the longest speech so far. The words were halting and spaced far apart, and even though he tried to hide the emotion behind them, his intensity was chilling.

"The only thing that bothers me is that every time I attach that bottle to my stomach tube, I feel like I'm watering a damned plant!"

I didn't know what to say, so I merely nodded and glanced down at the chart. If it had only been the lack of necessary tongue tissue, Tony probably could have managed liquids or soft food by mouth. Gravity would have been his ally. But the gunshot wound had destroyed his epiglottis, a small cartilage structure that sits over the entrance to the windpipe. Nature has designed it so that when swallowing occurs, it closes and prevents food from "going down the wrong way." As if

79

that weren't enough, one of Tony's vocal cords had been paralyzed by the injury, so the second safeguard that the body had provided, the closing of the vocal cords when swallowing, was also denied him. Anything Tony took by mouth would be inhaled, going into the windpipe and lungs, causing severe coughing spells.

Although I was overwhelmed with compassion, I tried not to show it, but he evidently sensed my feeling. "Well, I guess it's not so bad," he reassured me. "I get along okay. I just write on the blackboard fifty times a day 'It's a helluva lot better than being dead.' "

"Did they ever catch the guy who shot you?"

Vicky jumped in again. "Oh, sure. You know how determined the boys in blue are when a nut takes out one of their own. They got him. He drew a sentence of from five to seven. He'll be eligible for parole in a couple of months."

I completed the history and physical, seething with indignation. Who was going to parole Anthony Rocco from the misery that had been inflicted upon him?

By the time I'd finished my ten-minute scrub and entered the O.R., Mr. Dimitrios was properly draped and heavily sedated. The team of nurses was ready, but Dr. Burke was nowhere in sight.

This was a case that would necessitate both a skin flap and a skin graft — two different procedures. Where tissue has been lost and thickness is required to replace it for padding, flaps are used. A peninsula of skin and fat is rotated from an adjoining area and is sutured to cover the wound. The other end is left attached to the original site, to continue the circulation. The technique creates an open wound where the flap was taken, but it is a clean, shallow one that can be covered by a graft, a split-thickness piece of skin that is completely freed and taken from another part of the body. It's kind of like robbing Peter to pay Paul.

Unwilling to waste time, I anesthetized Mr. Dimitrios's heel and traced a triangle around the ulcer with a marking pen, indicating the tissue to be removed, then drew an adjacent oblong area, which would serve as the skin flap. Since the patient was lying on his stomach to make the heel operation easier, the back of his thigh was the logical donor site for the split-thickness skin graft needed to cover the original flap area. I anesthetized it with Xylocaine.

In light of the delay, I decided to check out the dermatome and make sure it was in proper working order. The dermatome is a marvelous device designed to cut a skin graft of uniform thickness. At University Hospital, we usually used a motor-driven type, which was equipped with a knife that moved back and forth like the blade of a haircutter. The thickness of the skin graft — from 0.001 to 0.030 of an inch — could be controlled by adjusting two calibrated knobs on either side, which altered the pitch of the blade. An attachment on either side gave us the desired width of the graft.

Obtaining skin grafts used to be a tedious and delicate procedure, done freehand by the plastic surgeon, using a long knife. Unfortunately, the quality of the graft varied greatly with the skill of the individual. The dermatome is one of the significant advances in our field.

There was nothing left to do now but the actual surgery, so I waited. Still no Dr. Burke. Knowing that another procedure was scheduled after ours in the O.R., I vacillated between waiting and going ahead. I had just opted for the latter when Dr. Burke puffed into the room. He was in a foul mood. Running his eyes over what I had done, he merely grunted and snatched a scalpel from the nurse's hand. The ulcer was deep, and his incision went almost to the bone. I reached for the electrocautery to assist with the bleeders, but he gestured me away angrily, and proceeded to deal with them himself. I inwardly shrugged, but, determined to be helpful, I extended my hand for a scalpel, intending to create the adjacent flap, so it could be rotated to cover the area where the ulcer had been.

"I'll do it, doctor," Burke said testily, making the flap himself and stitching it down.

I stood like an idiot, doing nothing except shifting my weight from one foot to the other, as Burke incised, sutured, tied, and cut. He personally took the skin graft and attached it to the new position. Finally, he straightened.

"All right, doctor," he said sarcastically, "the least you can do is the dressing. I'm running late." And with that he rushed from the room.

As I applied the bandage, I was burning with anger. Then reason prevailed and I realized that the past

hour had not been an utter waste of time. I had acquired information that later would be useful. From
the operating team, I learned that Burke was habitually ten to twenty minutes late. I discovered that he
was singularly unpopular with the O.R. staff. And now
I knew that as far as "our number two" man was concerned, I'd have to make an effort to look out for myself if I wanted the opportunity to "do" instead of
"observe." I was more than willing to match wits with
Dr. Alfred Burke, and I felt no guilt concerning my
uncharitable thoughts. One of his functions — one of
the services for which he was being paid — was to teach
me plastic surgery. The patients were not his private
domain. The resident training program decreed that I
should be doing part of every operation. I'd be
damned if I was going to sit around and let Burke
scoop up cases solely to refine his own techniques.

Now in a better mood, I made rounds — but I could
not stop thinking about Tony Rocco. The recollection
of that pleasant and courageous man's hand blocking
the trach tube each time he uttered a word, the image
of his being forced to feed himself three times a day
through a tube in his abdomen for the rest of his life,
haunted me. Instead of going to the doctors' lounge as
I usually did, I headed for University Hospital's huge
and very comprehensive medical library. Dr. Bob Sutton, the first-year resident who was assisting in the
clinic, was there studying. I needed a sounding board,
and I filled him in on the details of Tony Rocco's
problems.

"God, Bob," I ended, "there must be a solution. With all the new techniques and discoveries, maybe there's something that everybody's missed."

With the enthusiasm of the young and hopeful, we threw ourselves into pulling down research volumes, retrieving recent articles on head and neck injuries, searching out journals, poring over transcripts of lectures by experts in the field. We read everything of significance that had been written about the problem in the past few years. After concentrated effort, we reluctantly gave up. It was hard for us to admit that there was nothing, absolutely nothing, we could do to alleviate Tony Rocco's problems. Even though we often performed complicated reconstructive surgery, some situations were beyond solution. Defeated and frustrated, we said goodnight.

It was a little after seven-thirty when I arrived home. Patsy was setting the table and she greeted me with a warm kiss.

"I was out all afternoon," she said, "but I picked up some Chinese food. Okay?"

"Great."

I glanced at the table and felt soothed. Even though we'd be eating a meal of take-out food, candles spread a soft glow over the table, glinting off our wedding-present goblets of crystal. Tea was steeping in a bone china pot. Trust Patsy to understand what a welcome change such elegance was after the blood-and-guts atmosphere of the hospital.

As we sat down to plates heaped with almond

chicken, fried rice, and egg rolls, she asked, "Do you want to tell me about your day first, or should I tell you about mine?"

"It's up to you," I said magnanimously, but before she could speak, I launched into an account of the triumphs and frustrations I'd experienced. In a non-stop monologue I relived the mammoplasty, the face-lift, my irritation with Dr. Burke, my efforts on Tony Rocco's behalf, and even retold Lou Augustine's sickie joke. Patsy had just gone to the kitchen to replenish the teapot when the phone rang.

"Honey," I called as I hung up, "got to go. An emergency."

I picked up my coat and sprinted for the door. I heard her come in from the kitchen and turned to wave good-bye. For the first time during our marriage, I saw resentment, even anger, in her face. It surprised me. She'd always been completely understanding of the demands before.

All the way to the hospital, I brooded over her strange reaction, but as I entered the Emergency Room, I pushed it from my mind.

Dr. Babcock, the E.R. doctor on duty, gestured me to a bed in one of the curtained-off areas. The staff was already busy cleaning a profusely bleeding finger wound. The patient, a little boy, was only four months old, and his distraught mother hovered anxiously nearby. As soon as the mother saw me, the words came tumbling out.

"It all happened so fast, doctor," she blurted. "I'd

stopped in this pet store to get a flea collar for our beagle, and I had Billy in my arms. I propped him up over my shoulder while I was paying the cashier and somehow he poked his finger into a rabbit cage and . . . and, oh, God . . . one of them — one of them bit him."

I nodded and examined the child's ring finger. Most of the skin on the palm side, about one-third down from the tip of his finger, had been bitten away, and part of the fatty tissue beneath was gone, too. But one of the tendons was visible in the bottom of the wound, and it was uninjured.

"He's so little," his mother moaned. "I should have been watching him. Please, doctor, you can save his finger, can't you?"

"We'll certainly try," I reassured her. Then, excusing myself, I headed for a phone out of earshot and dialed Dr. Parmenter's exchange. Stitching the sailor's face wound the previous night had been routine, but this was a more complex situation, and I felt it advisable to check.

When Parmenter finally came on the line, I quickly filled him in on the injury. He listened until I'd finished.

"What procedure would you suggest?" he asked.

I had anticipated the question. In such injuries, there are two options, and I was prepared to defend my decision. I was fully aware that in the case of an adult, a skin flap would have been the preferred treatment. But it is an involved procedure necessitating several operations. With a child, I felt a full-thickness skin graft would be more desirable, and I said so to Dr. Parmenter.

"You're right," the Chief of Plastic Surgery agreed. Then he hesitated. "Look, Don, I'm tied up for a while." The sound of party noises in the background filtered through. "Do you want to call our number two man, or do you want to do it yourself?"

"No need to bother Dr. Burke," I said quickly. "Dr. Sutton's still here. He can assist."

"All right. If you have any problems, any problems at all, call me," Parmenter advised. "Then I'll come over."

I hung up with a feeling of satisfaction. I knew that most of the cases in plastic surgery did not require more advanced technical skill than I already had acquired from my four years in general surgery. It was not a case of a fledgling trying his wings; I was an experienced, adult bird, simply flying alone for the first time over slightly different terrain.

As Bob Sutton and I scrubbed, I briefly filled him in on the injury and the technique I intended to use. Then we both headed for the O.R.

Our little patient had been prepped and anesthetized. I took a small area of skin from the left groin, where the tiny scar wouldn't show, and carefully laid it on a wet sponge to keep it moist. The groin has extra folds of skin, and all that was necessary to close the wound was simple suturing. Then I turned my attention back to cleansing the finger wound with sterile saline solution. When I reached for the piece of skin, both it and the sponge had disappeared.

I searched around for a few moments. "Where's the skin for the graft?" I demanded. "I had it right here." Bob blinked several times. "Oh Jesus! Was it on the right corner of the tray?" I nodded. Bob gulped. "I — I passed it off the field with the other used sponges. I thought . . ." Mesmerized, everyone in the room gazed at the partially filled bucket of soiled gauze pads. The graft was contaminated, irretrievable.

There was a heavy silence as we glanced uncertainly at one another. I felt a momentary numbness. It was odd, but massive hemorrhage, shock, even cardiac arrest, would have geared us to instant action. We would have coped efficiently and quickly. Yet one tiny piece of missing skin left me dazed. What in hell were we to do now?

Barbara Fowler, our scrub nurse, was the first to recover. She glanced at me and began prepping the child's groin on the opposite side.

"You'll want to take another full thickness, won't you, doctor?" she said. "I'll have it ready for you in a minute."

Within moments I would have come up with the same solution, but I offered up a silent hosanna to each and every tactful, knowledgeable scrub nurse who, like Barbara, often rescues the pride of surgeons.

It was almost eleven when I got home, and Patsy was propped up in bed, reading. I hastened to make amends.

"Honey, I'm sorry about tonight. Gosh, I was so wound up during dinner, I didn't give you a chance to get a word in edgewise."

"So — what was the emergency?" she asked tartly, ignoring the apology.

Anxious not to compound my earlier error, I kept my reply short. "A baby — bitten by a rabbit."

To my bewilderment, Patsy's shoulders began to shake. At first I thought she was crying, but then I realized that she was convulsed with laughter. Noticing my baffled reaction, Patsy buried her face in the pillow, valiantly striving to suppress her mirth.

"Well, I don't see anything funny about a baby being bitten by a rabbit," I said, trying not to sound huffy. "But forget it. You said you were out all day. Who did you see?" My words only made her laugh harder. Slowly she rolled over to face me.

"That's what's so hysterical," she gasped. "I saw a rabbit about a baby. I had a doctor's appointment today. The test came up positive. Honey, I'm pregnant!"

Chapter Five

I WAS EUPHORIC at the prospect of being a father as I made early rounds Thursday, but by midmorning things started to go badly — and while I wouldn't have believed it possible, they became steadily worse.

Having seen our heel flap patient, Mr. Dimitrios, whose condition was excellent, I was surprised to be paged and told by the floor nurse that I'd better get up to his room as soon as possible.

As I have mentioned, Mr. Dimitrios was a victim of erratically fluctuating moods. When the sedation had worn off and he discovered himself alive, he was vaguely disappointed. So right after breakfast, he had called his wife, plus every member of his large family, summoning them to his bedside. Along with being capricious, Mr. Dimitrios was apparently very wealthy, and when the tribe was called, by God, they came running.

Entering the room, I became part of an unbelievable scene. I have never been able to determine exactly what Mr. Dimitrios told his family, but the tenor of it was that the surgeons had discovered some horrible, terminal condition — and had offered no hope of recovery. Maybe his alcoholism had done sufficient damage to cause irrationality, or perhaps he truly believed what he was saying, but I suspect Mr. Dimitrios was merely livening up an otherwise boring morning.

At any rate, my patient was sitting ramrod-straight in bed, castigating his family, concentrating particularly on his sons, yelling and pointing his finger as, one by one, he formally disowned them. The three men, all in their forties, were crushed; one was actually in tears. The two daughters were also distraught, although somewhat more in possession of their senses, because the ax of disinheritance hadn't yet fallen on their heads.

"I'm going to die!" Mr. Dimitrios thundered. "But none of you ingrates — not you — or you — are going to profit by it!"

A nurse was trying to restrain Mr. Dimitrios's wife. As I watched, she broke away and threw herself against the wall repeatedly, then finally flung herself on top of the patient.

"Nicholas, Nicholas," she screamed, "take me with you!"

I decided to step in. "Mr. Dimitrios is fine. He's not going anywhere except home — in about three days," I said. "And I'd suggest that all of you leave, right now. You're violating hospital visiting regulations."

I waited to make sure they left, and then followed them out. They besieged me with a dozen anxious questions. It was hard to convince them that Mr. Dimitrios's death was not imminent, and that they would have time to reinstate themselves in his good graces. I heard their father's voice petulantly calling me back to his side, and I expected a lecture from him about interfering with family matters. Instead, Mr. Dimitrios had docilely settled into his pillows.

"Where's the luncheon menu, doctor?" he complained plaintively. "I haven't filled out the slip for the diet kitchen yet. And I don't want fish again. You find out where it is, you hear?"

I was still shaking my head as I passed the nursing station. The girl who had been restraining Mrs. Dimitrios was holding a Kleenex against the back of her wrist.

"What happened to you?" I asked.

"The old biddy bit me," she announced.

I wanted to laugh, but it wasn't funny. Wounds from human bites are contaminated with a host of bacteria, and they can be dangerous. I examined the area and was relieved to note that Mrs. Dimitrios's teeth had barely opened the skin. Even so, the peril was there.

"I want you to go to Emergency right away," I ordered, "and have them clean and dress it. Be sure to tell them what happened so they'll give you a tetanus shot and antibiotics." She nodded.

"On the day you discharge Mr. Dimitrios," she sighed, "I'll buy you a drink."

I had only progressed a few steps before I was paged again. This time Miss Farrell passed along the information that I was to join Dr. Parmenter in his office for a consultation with another surgeon.

My boss was popular and had an outstanding reputation among the other staff physicians at University Hospital. He was knowledgeable in the field of head and neck cancers, and Dr. Avery Jackson, an Ear, Nose and Throat specialist, had asked his assistance on a case currently in the Intensive Care Unit.

They quickly filled me in. The patient was Colonel John Bainbridge. Over the past year, Dr. Jackson had performed three major operations on him for a neck malignancy that had started in a salivary gland. But the cancer had recurred, and the question was "What do we do now?"

"The damn thing's sitting right over the carotid artery," Jackson groaned, "and it's bound to invade it."

The carotid artery is the largest in the neck. Once the malignant cells penetrated, the patient would start to bleed, and he would bleed to death. There would be no stopping it.

"Of course, I'll want to examine him," Parmenter said, "but as you say, I imagine the only hope is to clamp the carotid artery and cut off the blood flow. Naturally, it will significantly increase the possibility of a stroke complication, but —"

Dr. Jackson nodded morosely. "We'll simply hope it doesn't happen. I just wanted a second opinion. John and I were in the army together, and I'm terribly fond of him and his wife. We're good friends. They've been my patients for years."

"Are you pleading personal involvement?" Parmenter asked gently. Often physicians, if they feel their closeness to a patient might impair their judgment, delegate the care to another physician. It is the primary reason why doctors refuse to minister to their immediate families.

"Not officially," Dr. Jackson hedged, "but I would appreciate it if you'd act as consultant and do the procedure." Parmenter graciously nodded. "If you have time to see the colonel now," Jackson suggested, "I'll go with you. His wife is upstairs, and I'd like you to meet her."

"Fine," Dr. Parmenter said. "Don, could you come along?"

Mrs. Bainbridge was waiting in the I.C.U. lounge. She had apparently been a beautiful woman, but age had been unkind. Now she was elderly, wan, and extremely nervous. After we'd been introduced, Dr. Parmenter urged her to sit down and, with his unlimited charm, was able to draw her out.

"It's been so very difficult, doctor," she said softly. "My husband — well, I want him home with me, but the tumor is so painful he won't even let me change the dressing. Dr. Jackson prescribed Demerol and taught me to give John the injections, but even though he's in agony, he absolutely refuses them." She turned to Dr. Jackson. "Avery, I can't stand to see him suffer. I just can't. When he gets home, you're going to have to *command* him to let me give him the shots. If he receives a direct order from you, he'll follow it."

"I will, dear, I will," Jackson assured her. I admired his gentleness, but from what I had heard so far, it was unlikely that Colonel Bainbridge would ever go home.

"With Mrs. Bainbridge, the colonel's pride makes him quite a handful," Dr. Jackson went on. "But in the hospital, he's entirely different. The staff considers him an ideal patient. He never complains. He takes care of himself as much as possible. He spent thirty-four years in the army, and loved every minute of it. He's been retired for eight years, and I honestly believe he likes the regimentation here. I think he finds it comforting."

Parmenter nodded. "It's highly possible. I'd like to examine your husband, Mrs. Bainbridge. Why don't you wait here?"

We picked up the colonel's chart and headed for his bed. He was crisply polite as I removed the dressing over the large ulcer, just below his right ear, that the tumor had created. One glance confirmed that it was infected and painful.

"I've ordered fresh antiseptic dressings four times a day," Jackson murmured. "I've also prescribed morphine every three hours for relief."

"Good," Parmenter agreed. He turned to me. "Don, see if you can clear a minor surgery room."

Shortly after that, under local anesthesia, we had made a small slit below the tumor, exposing the carotid artery, which, fortunately, lies not far beneath the

95

skin. A Silverstone clamp, a tiny rectangular hinged vise, was placed around the artery, and the screw was left protruding through the skin so that it could be turned, causing a vertical closing in direct relationship to the number of revolutions. Our plan was to tighten the Silverstone clamp a little every day, so that the artery would be closed gradually, rather than suddenly. We hoped this would minimize the probability of a stroke. We all realized that the clamp would do nothing to treat the basic problem, the tumor itself. It was only a means of preventing a massive hemorrhage and death within minutes if — no, when — the carcinoma ate into the carotid artery. Colonel Bainbridge's condition was incurable and, sooner or later, he was going to die because of it.

"Let's watch him like a hawk, Don," Parmenter instructed. "Any symptoms of hypertension and we'll just back off . . . loosen the clamp a little . . . and see what happens."

While I held on to the satisfaction of knowing that we were doing all we could, still I had not learned to accept defeat gracefully. I never would. Inevitable death was a personal affront. Once the patient had been wheeled out and was on his way back to the I.C.U., I voiced my frustration.

"It was an interesting procedure," I said dejectedly, "but all we're doing is buying time. There isn't a shred of hope, is there?"

"Don't ever ask me that," Dr. Parmenter said softly. "We win some . . . we lose some."

I was debating the merits of an early lunch when I received the information that Mr. and Mrs. Harris had arrived and that George, their seven-month-old son, had been admitted. Dr. Burke had seen the child previously and had scheduled him for surgery in the morning — but, the nurse reported, the little boy was spiking a fever of 100.6 degrees. Could I take a look?

Once on the floor, I scanned the patient's chart. Little George had been born with a skin growth on his upper left arm, and it had become progressively larger. Biopsies had been done earlier and a small piece of tissue from the area had been examined under the microscope by the pathologists. As sometimes happens, there was a difference of opinion. One contingent thought it was a juvenile melanoma. These are not terribly serious, but it is thought that they can become malignant, and although most simple skin cancers are easily treated by local surgical removal, excising a malignant melanoma is an operation of much greater magnitude.

Others of the pathologists had diagnosed the growth as a giant hairy pigmented nevus. Although this is only essentially a mole with hair growing from it, the area it covers can be considerable.

Whatever it was, removal had been recommended, and even though no one was anxious to operate on a seven-month-old, all agreed that the situation warranted it.

According to Burke's notes, he intended to remove a large portion of the lesion and cover the area with a skin graft from the baby's back. To minimize the trauma, the remainder of the growth would be removed some months later. But the fever, if it persisted, would mean canceling tomorrow's surgery.

I entered the room and introduced myself to the Harrises. Both were only eighteen years old and extremely immature. Amy Harris cradled her child almost defiantly as she paced back and forth. Her husband, Jimmy, sat wide-eyed in a chair, biting his fingernails. The nurse who had followed me in took George from a reluctant Mrs. Harris and laid the tot on the bed, removing the thin blanket that had been covering him.

While I was in medical school, giant hairy nevus cases had been grouped with other congenital deformities and had been touched upon, but somewhat lightly. They were comparatively rare, and I'd never actually encountered one before. So when I began my examination, I was totally unprepared for what I saw. From the top of the child's shoulder, down past the elbow, was a heavy sheath of hair — dense, black, shiny, the strands two to three inches long — literally a sleeve. Esthetically, it was hideous. When I was a kid, I had explored my grandmother's attic and had come across a monkey fur jacket. I couldn't help being struck by the resemblance.

The nurse took George's temperature again. It hadn't changed — still 100.6. I indicated the tests I wanted done to try to pinpoint the source of the fever, and she hurried out. Before I'd finished my examination, a lab technician appeared to draw blood.

Whether I was forewarned by instinct or my previous experience on the pediatrics ward, I sensed imminent trouble. I turned to Mr. and Mrs. Harris.

"I'm going to be here for a while," I said cheerfully; "why don't you go have a cup of coffee?"

In unison they shook their heads. Shrugging, I nodded to the technician to proceed. No one likes having a needle stuck into them; naturally the baby began to cry.

Mrs. Harris became unglued.

"Stop it," she shrieked; "you're hurting him!" She grasped the technician's arm. "Just stop it!"

"Mrs. Harris," I said, leading her away, "your son has a fever, and we're trying to find out why. Unless we can get it down, the surgery tomorrow will have to be postponed." Her eyes widened and she sank heavily into a chair. The lab man was able to draw the blood without further interference.

"Take it easy," I urged the young couple. "We'll wait and see. I'll check with you after lunch."

I had just reached the head of a considerable line in the cafeteria when I heard myself paged. There was a problem with the Harrises, and I went back upstairs.

Amy Harris was standing in the hall in hysterics, tears streaming down her cheeks, announcing to everyone who passed — patients, nurses, visitors, doctors — that her child had inoperable cancer.

I tried to reassure her. George did *not* have cancer. The *only* thing that would prevent surgery was her child's fever. She barely listened.

"I know it's cancer," she screeched. "A biopsy was

99

taken, wasn't it? And you take biopsies for cancer! Can you operate or not?"

"I don't know yet." I felt like an idiot. A group of visitors had paused en route to their destinations, and had formed about us. The pathetic sight of this distraught young mother couldn't help evoking sympathy. I suddenly realized that her accusing questions had been strident; my words of explanation had been audible only to her.

"Every minute counts, and you don't care!" she gasped. "You don't care if my baby dies!" Glancing at the people around us, I decided on the best course of action — to get the hell away from there as fast as I could.

"I'll check back with you later this afternoon," I called.

Too late for any lunch now. It was almost three, and I could picture the patients jamming the Plastic Surgery Outpatient Clinic.

I changed into a fresh tunic and went out to the desk to summon the first patient. The stack of charts was slightly askew and I paused to straighten them, feeling Miss Farrell's eyes on me all the time. I knew she resented my compulsiveness, but something within me always screamed for order.

For instance, on the left side of the bathroom vanity in our apartment, *my* hairbrush and comb were *always* laid precisely perpendicular. It was a running gag. Whenever Patsy came in while I was shaving, in passing she'd slightly move one or the other and then smile as, subsconsciously, my hand reached out to move them back into perfect alignment.

I met Miss Farrell's eyes and shrugged, slightly embarrassed. On the other hand, if I ever needed a surgeon myself, I'd rather he be compulsive than haphazard.

My eyes skimmed over the top chart before I picked it up. Mrs. Weinstein, with her three-year-old son, Benny. I read no further, but allowed my gaze to roam the room. In a far corner sat a woman desperately trying to control what I judged was a hyperactive little boy. Her eyes were red-rimmed and her sniffling could be heard throughout the reception area. I was not up to coping with another distraught mother and problem child at that moment. Dr. Bob Sutton appeared behind me, ready to start, and I casually handed the top chart to him, feeling a twinge of guilt as the woman and child followed him in. I picked up the next chart. Mrs. Frederick Baynes, forty-one years old. I called out the name and was vastly relieved when an exceptionally well-dressed, composed woman arose. I asked her to proceed to the examining room, and paused for a moment to fill in Miss Farrell about the Harris child's complication.

"I'll inform Dr. Burke," she said, frowning. For the second time, I had the feeling conveyed to me that the little boy's problems were somehow my fault. Damn and double damn!

When I reached the examining room I found Mrs. Baynes seated on the table. She had removed her blouse and bra and the nurse had given her a sheet, which she was now clutching around her upper torso for dear life. It was not unusual. Most patients are normally modest. But she was trembling.

"I'm Dr. Moynihan, one of the plastic surgeons here," I began as usual. "Whatever your problem is, maybe I can help."

"My breasts . . . ," she whispered.

I waited expectantly for her to go on. Were they too small or too large? With the sheet enveloping her, it was impossible to tell. She continued to stare at me and I sensed rising panic.

"Mrs. Baynes," I said gently, "I'm going to have to examine you."

Reluctantly — ever so reluctantly — she removed the sheet. Her breasts were purplish, misshapen, and badly infected. Visible lumps were everywhere, and there were multiple oozing and open sores of various sizes where the skin had begun ulcerating. One nipple was putrefied almost to the point of dropping off.

Tijuana silicone rot! I'd seen cases of it before.

The medical profession is painfully aware that there are several prosperous surgeons who practice just across the border in Mexico, who've become millionaires by doing breast augmentations. Injecting industrial grade raw silicone directly into the tissue, they use a cheap commercial material that sells for about fifteen dollars a gallon and is manufactured as a base for floor waxes, polishes, electrical insulation, and water-repellent sprays. In recent years, over five hundred cases have been treated by legitimate doctors in and near the large cities in Southern California. The process is, of course, outlawed in the United States.

"I take it you had silicone shots in Mexico," I said. "How long ago?"

"About two years," she managed to reply. "I answered an advertisement in a 'personals' column of one of the newspapers. My breasts have always been small and . . . Anyway, the ad promised 'Beautiful Busts Without Surgery,' so I answered it. I was told to drive to a place in the city, where a woman — she said she was a nurse — met me and drove us across the border to a doctor's office in Tijuana. He promised that his treatments worked, and that it was no more unpleasant than a series of vitamin shots. Altogether, he gave me eight injections."

"What did he charge you?"

"A little over eight hundred dollars."

I tried to keep the wonderment out of my face. "Mrs. Baynes! For a few hundred dollars more, you could have had a legitimate surgeon here perform the implant operation."

"Oh I know that."

"Then why go to Mexico?"

She lowered her eyes. "I didn't want anyone cutting on me. I'm terrified of surgery. Down there it seemed so simple — and quick — and —"

Simple and quick. Except for the aftereffects. It is officially estimated that seventy percent of the women who cross the border for the breast-building injections will eventually have serious, occasionally life-threatening, complications. Some feel the figure is too conservative — that a hundred percent is more realistic. And the consequences are ugly. The raw silicone sometimes migrates through the bloodstream to the brain, the lungs, and the heart, with the risk of blindness, strokes, gangrene, and a variety of other organic troubles, sometimes ending in death. Because the appropriate Mexican laws are loose and enforcement is lax, there has been little success in curbing the activity. Nor can any legal action be taken against the women employed as recruiters.

"Everything was fine until just recently," Mrs. Baynes volunteered. "Then I started having terrible pain, so I went back to Mexico on my own to see the doctor. He gave me a shot of cortisone and told me to stop worrying. But it got worse. I went back a few weeks ago, and he said there was nothing he could do."

I sighed.

"You can help me, doctor, can't you?" she asked.

"I'll try, Mrs. Baynes, but I think I should be honest with you. We'll concentrate on trying to save the breast skin. If that works, we can surgically remove the tissue and the standard augmentation mammoplasty *might* be possible."

"*If* it works?" she repeated apprehensively.

It had to be said, and there wasn't any easy way. "Your skin is in pretty bad shape." She started to cry, and my heart went out to her. "We'll hope for the best.

In any event, there's a lot we *can* do. I'll want to see you back here in two days. In the meantime —"

I wrote her a prescription for oral antibiotics and explained that I wanted her to try what we call wet-to-dry dressings. Gauze pads soaked in a saline solution are applied and not removed until they have dried. They adhere to the wound and when the dressing is pulled off, it takes dead tissue with it. It is a means of cleaning the wounds. The magnitude of Mrs. Baynes's infection made minor surgery inevitable. The nipple would have to be removed and the dead tissue cut away. It could be done as an outpatient procedure, with little or no anesthesia, since dead tissue is insensitive. I made a mental note to schedule it for the next time I saw her, but didn't mention it. Mrs. Baynes was going through enough agony at the moment.

After she left, I sat in a nearby chair to muster my thoughts.

Until recently, augmentation mammoplasties with the preformed silicone gel sacs had been designed and used mainly for cosmetic purposes. But, as with all medical breakthroughs, the possibility for other uses — such as breast restoration — had become excitingly apparent.

Take women with chronic cystic mastitis. There are many females who, for reasons unknown, suffer a seemingly never-ending series of benign breast cysts. Yet, with each lump discovered, a biopsy must be performed to make sure the pattern hasn't changed — that the new mass isn't malignant. Normally, the physician will attempt to aspirate the lump. If he is successful in withdrawing fluid with a needle and if the cyst disappears within a short time, he can be sure of his diagnosis of nonmalignancy. But occasionally that technique fails. Then the patient must be hospitalized for a surgical biopsy. Even though the cyst is discovered to be benign, she is forced to undergo the agony of waiting for the dreaded pathologist's report, signing the operative release for the surgeon to proceed with a mastectomy if the news is bad, wondering if she'll be whole or mutilated when she awakens, and coping with the ever increasing cost of frequent hospitalizations. I've known women who've developed new lumps every few months, year after year — and their lives are lived under an umbrella of fear.

Others suffer from mastodynia, a painful condition caused by clogged ducts that recurs again and again.

Until recently, the only alternative was the amputation of both breasts, a rather radical procedure for a benign disease. Now women with these difficulties have the option of a subcutaneous mastectomy, a relatively new operation that is being done more frequently as public awareness increases. The procedure involves the removal of the cyst-producing gland tissue, but leaves the breast skin and nipples intact. Implants are inserted, restoring the breast form. There can be complications, but I personally feel it is worth the risk for women who are constantly developing new lumps that can't be distinguished from cancer.

An even newer plastic surgery procedure permits,

under certain conditions, the rebuilding of a breast after a malignancy-necessitated mastectomy. When you realize that eventually five and nine-tenths percent of women, one out of every seventeen, will develop breast cancer, this most recent innovation is very significant. There are limitations. Four different mastectomy procedures are recognized, ranging from simply cutting out the cancerous lump — popularly known as a "lumpectomy" — to the radical operation in which the entire breast is removed, along with the two main chest muscles and the lymph nodes in the armpit. In between there are techniques called "simple" and "modified radical" mastectomies, depending on how much tissue is removed. Faced with cancer, the general surgeon is chiefly concerned with saving the patient's life, and the type of operation he elects to do is governed by the tumor's size and location, and the patient's history. Cosmetic considerations must remain secondary. Now, however, following all but the most "radical" procedure, where the pectoralis muscles are removed, it is sometimes possible to reconstruct the breast with a silicone implant.

Some general surgeons are beginning to discuss this option with their mastectomy patients. Unfortunately, many are not. Perhaps they can't fully understand the horror that most women feel about such mutilation. A few have the attitude that the patient's life has been saved . . . she should be grateful . . . what more does she want? Admittedly, the reconstruction procedure is fairly new, expensive, and relatively complicated, and sometimes the end result leaves much to be desired. Another consideration is that since the size of the prosthesis is limited by the breast skin available, often reduction mammoplasty is required on the other breast to attain symmetry.

On the plus side, however, there is no danger of stirring up dormant cancer cells, nor does the implant interfere with future physical examination for possible recurrence. And, when it works, the emotional rewards are tremendous. The restoration removes the visible reminder of the dreaded bout with Big C. The patient can get dressed and undressed without feeling sorry for herself. Embarrassment during sexual encounters is lessened. Still, the new technique is not a panacea. Many women are unacceptable candidates for the reconstructive surgery. But it's worth inquiring about. Those who successfully undergo the operation are handed a new lease on life.

When she went out, Mrs. Baynes had left the door slightly ajar, and my thoughts were interrupted as Dr. Sutton poked in his head.

"Aha," he said. "Goofing off!"

"Just trying to get it all together," I said. "You wouldn't believe the day I've had." He started to leave, and I called him back. "Bob? That Mrs. Weinstein and her son Benny — what was the problem?"

He paused, remembering. "Oh, Mrs. Weinstein is afraid that Benny is going to have a hooked nose like his father. She wanted it fixed. I explained that we

don't do rhinoplasties until the bone quits growing."
He grinned. "She's going to call back for another
appointment — in about thirteen years."

"Why was she crying?"

"Crying?" He puzzled on that for a moment. "Oh,
she wasn't crying. She's got an allergy — to lemon blos-
soms, I think."

As Dr. Sutton shut the door, I realized that in the
manipulated patient exchange, I'd gotten the worst of
the bargain.

The rest of the clinic cases were pretty much run-of-
the-mill. I was not on call that night, thank goodness,
because I was really strung out — and once I'd finished
up, I decided that instead of hanging around as I normally did, I'd go home. And I was glad I did.

The saga of the Harrises and their son George continued, and since Dr. Burke made evening rounds instead of me, he bore the brunt of it. The child's temperature was still up, and none of the tests ordered had
been able to pinpoint the cause. In infants, this is not
terribly rare. "F.U.O." — fever of unknown origin —
was a notation that regularly popped up on the charts.
Unless other symptoms appear, standard procedure is
to wait it out. But when Burke went into the room,
Mr. and Mrs. Harris were still cemented in their
chairs, and according to what I heard later, Mrs. Harris
looked terrible — flushed and hardly able to talk.
Burke discovered that she was running a temperature,
too, and sent her to the Emergency Room. She made
quite a fuss there, complaining of a terribly stiff neck,

which turned out to be an infected throat. But the E.R. doctor, intimidated by her dramatics, suspected meningitis and did a spinal tap. It turned out negative, but unfortunately Mrs. Harris developed a spinal headache from the procedure. This is not serious, but it is extremely bothersome. The patient must lie flat and drink lots of fluids. Assuming an upright position brings the pain rushing back.

At any rate, an argument erupted between Mrs. Harris and Dr. Burke. He began by suggesting she go home; she refused. He pointed out that her infection might endanger the child; she countered inanely by reminding him that she was George's mother. Finally, he banished her from the room, expecting that this would make her go home. Later, he found her lying on a couch in the family room. Nothing but physical force would dislodge her, and Dr. Burke simply gave up and fled.

Early in the morning, when he made rounds, she was still there, and he had to tell her that because of the child's sustained fever, the anesthesiologists had canceled George's surgery. She had hysterics again. Burke tried logic. Although the surgery was necessary, it certainly wasn't an emergency. Mrs. Harris's weeping drowned further attempts at explanation. Luckily, at this point, Miss Farrell was passing in the corridor, on her way to meet Parmenter. She listened for a moment and took over.

"Just knock it off," she commanded. Mrs. Harris's eyes widened and her tantrum ceased instantly. Miss

Farrell extended the clipboard that was practically a part of her. "Now, write down your mother's phone number." Mrs. Harris took the pencil and obediently scribbled the information. Within an hour, George's grandmother and grandfather had arrived to take them all home. Why hadn't anyone else thought of that? Fortunately, the grandparents turned out to be much more sensible than the others and were entirely satisfied when the reason for the delayed surgery was explained. So, with a sigh of relief, Dr. Burke signed the discharge order, and the Harrises disappeared, at least for the time being.

Chapter Six

OUTPATIENT MINOR SURGERY was scheduled each Friday morning, and I joined Dr. Burke there. His adventures with the Harrises had not improved his disposition, and I had the feeling it was going to be a long morning.

Our first operation was on a young man by the name of Schenck — Peter Schenck. His problem was strictly cosmetic — he felt that his lips were too prominent, and I had to agree. I stood and watched as Dr. Burke anesthetized the area and removed an ellipse of tissue and a substantial amount of underlying fat from the inside of Pete's lips. I doubted that such a simple procedure could give a good result but, as it turned out, it worked. Mr. Schenck's lips were considerably reduced in size and had a more normal appearance. Score one for Dr. Burke.

Our next patient was a young man with a tattoo on his upper arm that he wanted removed — a large multicolored eagle perched on a waving American flag. Dr. Burke had a habit of disappearing for long periods between procedures, and I had a chance to talk to Michael Cranston. It was the usual story. He'd been in the marines and, after a night of drinking, he and his buddies decided to top off the evening with a trip to a tattoo shop. These "artists" are usually strategically wedged between bars and massage parlors, ready to prey on the drunk and the dim-witted. After the war, Cranston had resumed his studies, received his teaching degree, and was doing well in his profession. But the tattoo was now an embarrassment. When he was golfing he wore a longsleeved shirt and avoided showering in the locker rooms. At pool parties, he pretended he was extremely sensitive to sunburn and lolled around fully clothed. Finally, tired of the charade, Mr. Cranston wanted the eagle emblem removed.

Rather than coming to a plastic surgeon years after having the tattoo applied, I wish the Mr. Cranstons of the world would give a little thought to the consequences beforehand, but I suppose that's a forlorn hope.

The eagle and flag extended over an area about two inches wide and some four inches high. Because of the size of the tattoo, I assumed that Burke intended to remove it entirely and use a skin graft replacement. As a general surgeon, I had treated tattoos this way and found it to be satisfactory. However, Dr. Burke disagreed. He insisted that it could be cut out and stitched up without a graft. He intended to remove the central portion of the tattoo today and do the rest at a future date, when the normal elasticity of the skin was restored.

I didn't agree with him, and out of earshot of the patient, we argued about it. But Burke was adamant and I had to yield. Burke removed a section of skin about five and a half inches long and an inch wide, going right through the middle of the eagle. He had to undermine much of the skin on each side to make it lax enough so that the edges would come together, and it took a great many stitches to keep the wound closed. As I suspected, this created tautness in the upper arm. I sure as hell didn't like the effect, but there was nothing to be done about it at that point. I decided, however, that in the future, whether or not I might be wrong and Dr. Burke might be right, if I had doubts, I'd appeal to Parmenter for a final opinion. That much I owed the patients.

The end result was amusing in a bizarre way. The midsection of the tattoo had been removed, and when the skin was closed, the head of the eagle was stitched to its tail.

I tried a feeble witticism. "Congratulations, Dr. Burke," I whispered. "You managed to change an eagle into a pigeon."

"Mr. Cranston will be fine," Burke said. "I only hope you can say the same about the kid with the rabbit bite that you and Dr. Sutton handled. I understand he's spiking a fever." And our "number two man" stalked away.

I squirmed because it was true. Little Billy Sweeny had been fine yesterday, but this morning he was running a temperature of 103 degrees. I'd ordered a workup to investigate the cause. A chest X-ray would determine if he had a partial collapse of the lung, which sometimes occurs after an operation, but it was highly unlikely in a four-month-old infant.

I'd also ordered some cultures of the blood and urine, but I knew that fever from a wound infection normally didn't show up for four or five days. To add to my frustration, I had tried to call Mrs. Sweeny to give her a progress report and had found out that the child's mother had refused to leave her residence telephone number, saying that she did not care to be disturbed at home. She had left an office number where she worked, but it was too early to get an answer. I was angry. It seemed to me that a mother with a four-month-old infant in the hospital suffering from a significant hand injury shouldn't mind a telephone call from the doctor about how her kid was doing.

By the time the minor surgery clinic was over, I would have the test results back on the baby. I just prayed that the skin graft would not be rejected. I didn't need that complication with my first solo operation on this service.

Our final case of the morning was a hair transplant operation on Mr. Elmer Tanner. This was his third series of hair plugs, and again Burke's absence allowed me to chat with our patient.

Mr. Tanner had just spent a solid year at a remote weather installation in Antarctica. When he'd kissed his wife good-bye and left the U.S.A., he'd had a good head of curly hair; when he'd returned, his hairline had receded and he had a sizable bald area in front. For some reason, this was a tremendous shock and a source of embarrassment to his wife. She wasn't about to let her friends and neighbors see Elmer bald, and she'd been nagging him to have a hair transplant. She'd had a face-lift two years ago and shortly thereafter a "tummy-tuck" operation. She bragged that she was a "new woman." Evidently she had decided to have her husband done over as well.

Mr. Tanner was ready and willing — so why not? Hair transplants have been performed for over twenty years. There have been few reports of failure. The procedure is somewhat tedious for both surgeon and patient, but it's simple enough.

With a circular scalpel, plugs are taken from the hair-bearing areas at the back or sides of the scalp and transplanted where needed. Mr. Tanner had what is called male-pattern baldness, with the front and crown areas affected. During the first session, a row of plugs had been transplanted from elsewhere on his head to the front to establish a hairline. That done, we'd worked back, spacing plugs until all of the area was covered. In order for the hair-bearing graft to be put in place, a matching circle in the recipient area is removed by the punch graft scalpel and discarded. Then the new plug is inserted. Stitching isn't necessary, for the grafts are held in place by a dressing. It isn't even necessary to close the donor sites, for within a few days they contract and heal quite nicely. When this procedure is done correctly, the loss of hair in the donor areas is unnoticeable. Usually about sixty plugs are transplanted at one time, separated enough to insure scalp circulation. Then in subsequent sessions, usually six weeks apart, additional plugs are placed between the initial ones until sufficient density is obtained.

To cover a large bald area, up to four hundred plugs may be needed, so five or six sessions are scheduled. Except for the injection of the Novocain, very little pain is involved. We are always careful to explain to the patient that he will never get more hair on his head than is already there. We simply move hair from one spot to another. Interestingly enough, a transplanted area will never again grow bald. The final result is never absolutely normal, but by combing and intermingling the natural hair with the transplants, you could fool anyone but an expert.

Dr. Burke finally arrived and we proceeded with the transplants.

As soon as the last plug was inserted, he muttered something about "being late" and dashed from the room. Even though I knew Mr. Tanner had undergone the procedure twice before, I reminded him that although the hairs in the donor grafts might appear to be growing the first month, they were really falling out. He should not expect true hair growth for about three months.

"I know, doc, I know."

Our would-be Samson took off with a genial wave,

and I headed upstairs for little Billy Sweeny's room. Dr. Parmenter happened to be in the corridor and we studied the test results.

"Have you changed the dressing on the finger yet?" Dr. Parmenter asked.

I shook my head. "I was just on my way."

"Good. I'll go with you and take a look."

Once the bandage was removed, we discovered Billy's finger was badly infected — swollen, red, and tender. We drained it and administered an antibiotic.

"I'd bet the fever is gone within twelve hours," the Chief commented.

"Damn," I replied, "you know, I thought about a wound infection and discarded the idea. I haven't seen all that many animal bites. If I'd just taken a look, I could have saved a lot of tests."

Parmenter shrugged. "Well, that's what you're here for — to learn."

He was right. Lectures or textbooks are great — but nothing beats actual experience. I wrote an order for the child's hand to be soaked for twenty minutes four times a day. The nurse took the chart, glanced at it, and sighed. That one line meant a full hour and a half of nursing time each day, for with a child as little as Billy, someone would have to be assigned to hold the hand in the sterile solution.

"Were you able to reach the child's mother, doctor?" the nurse asked.

My lips tightened as I reached for the phone. "No," I said shortly. "I'll try again. Now she's probably out to lunch!" At Dr. Parmenter's questioning look, I filled him in. My distaste for a mother who cared so little about her kid came through.

"Don," Parmenter said casually, "why don't you wait until you run into Mrs. Sweeny during visiting hours? I know it bugs you not to be able to get in touch with her at home, but maybe she has a good reason." He paused. "Billy's going to be okay — besides, we're not here to ride herd on the dingbats of the world."

A little put out, I hung up before I'd completed dialing. Later I would discover that Mrs. Sweeny lived in a panic-engulfed world. She was divorced from her husband and living with another man. Her "ex" was vindictive, and twice he'd inflicted bodily harm upon her. He didn't really want Billy, but he was harassing Mrs. Sweeny unmercifully and taking every legal step possible to get custody of the child. Mrs. Sweeny lived in terror at the thought of anyone discovering she was "living in sin" and of being declared unfit. Remembering the genuine anguish of the woman when she'd brought her son in, I knew that my irritation at her apparent lack of concern had been misdirected. Two lessons learned: don't overlook the obvious, and until you're sure, don't embrace what seems obvious as fact.

I looked in on Mr. Dimitrios. His heel flap was mending splendidly and I signed a discharge order. He could go home tomorrow. I was just about to leave his room when I heard myself paged. I picked up the bedside phone and flashed the operator, who was holding a call for me from the Emergency Room.

"We have a burn case, doctor," the nurse informed me tersely. "Are you available?"

"I'll be right down."

I've mentioned the competition between the various medical services for cases. But one thing is certain, and you'd better believe it — there is *never* a fight over burn patients. Requiring an intensive period of acute care and long-term treatment after the critical stage, a severe burn is a truly miserable situation — and nobody battles for the responsibility.

I remember one evening when I was serving my general surgery residency. I had gone to the Intensive Care Unit to check on another patient and noticed a man lying in an adjacent bed. He was sixty-seven years old and had been brought into the Emergency Room the night before with major burns over fifty percent of his body. There was no medical history. Evidently he had been found in a tenement apartment that had caught fire. His injuries included one hundred percent burn of the face, neck, and head. His left arm and leg, both feet, and his entire back were horribly charred. Everything possible had been done, but he'd been in shock since admission, and his life was hanging by a thread. The odor was overwhelming. It was hard to realize that this was a human being — a human being who had laughed, listened to the radio, gone to the supermarket, perhaps begotten children. A smoldering cigarette, a pan of grease left too long on a stove, or maybe a frayed electric cord had transformed him into a cinder.

The next morning, when I'd stopped in the I.C.U., the bed was empty. I didn't have to ask to know that he'd died. For a while, I couldn't get it out of my mind. Then, a few days later, I happened to see pictures in the newspaper of a fire in a high-rise building in New Orleans. The blaze had broken out on the twenty-first or twenty-second floor and everyone above had been trapped. When it became certain that they were cut off with no hope of rescue, six of the occupants jumped from the windows of the building. The news photographer's lens had vividly caught the reaction of the screaming crowds below as they watched the horrifying drama of human beings deliberately flinging themselves to their death. Yet, after seeing the man in Intensive Care, I wondered if I might not do the same in a similar situation.

As I made my way to the Emergency Room, I hoped it might be a minor injury. No such luck. The patient was a four-year-old girl who had received third-degree burns from the knees to the ankles, and second-degree burns of the lower thighs.

The skin is made up of two layers. The epidermis is the thin outer protective layer. It's the part that peels after a sunburn. The majority of the skin's thickness is dermis, which contains hair follicles, sweat glands, nerves, and blood vessels. First-degree burns are characterized by redness and swelling of the skin, and involve only the epidermis. They usually require no therapy except for relief of pain. Second-degree burns, with blister formation and weeping, destroy the epidermis and a portion of the dermis. They sometimes heal with minimum scarring if infection can be avoided. Third-degree burns destroy the full thickness of the skin and often involve the underlying tissue as well, and unless these areas are very small they must be skin-grafted.

The patient's mother was too upset to talk, so the nurse filled me in. Mrs. Hancock had invited some of the neighborhood children to play with her daughter, Donna. Planning a wiener roast for them, she'd started a fire in the backyard barbecue that her husband had built, then had dashed inside to get buns and Cokes and paper plates. In those few minutes, Donna had somehow climbed up on the piece of corrugated aluminum that served as the roof of the barbecue pit. The sheeting collapsed and she slid, feet first, into the white-hot charcoal briquettes. Immobilized with terror, Donna had been unable to move until, just seconds later, her screams had brought her mother on the run to pull her out. But by then, the child's slacks had caught fire and the flesh of her legs was sizzling.

To save time, the Emergency Room had recruited an anesthesiologist, who had given Donna an injection of ketamine and had started an IV. With that done, my first order of business was to make sure that the swelling of the burned tissue didn't cut circulation to the lower legs and feet.

So, taking up a scalpel, I made long vertical incisions through the skin on both sides of the lower legs. An incision in burned tissue is called an escharotomy, and the principle is that when significant swelling from the burns begins, these skin edges will just open up and pull apart, preventing the skin from forming a constricting band. When the edema goes down, the long incisions heal up surprisingly well without even being closed with sutures. Third-degree burns, oddly enough, are not very painful, for the nerve endings have been destroyed.

Ketamine, the anesthetic which had been given, is very effective but it occasionally causes children to become hyperactive and sometimes to hallucinate. This happened with Donna. Once I'd completed the escharotomy, she began thrashing about, and the IV needle that had been inserted came out. I quickly had her transferred to the Intensive Care Unit so I could get a cut-down catheter in place with minimum time loss. A "cut-down" is essentially an intravenous line that is surgically placed by making an incision, usually in the arm or leg, and exposing a suitable vein. Its value is that instead of relying on a small needle, a good sized catheter can be secured in the vein with stitches. The inevitable swelling that accompanies burns is caused by great quantities of fluid rushing to the injured area. This seriously depletes the circulating fluid volume, and it is absolutely crucial that large amounts of water and other solutions be delivered in the first eight to twelve hours after the injury to replace what has been lost; otherwise, the patient may die of shock.

Let me tell you, you haven't lived until you attempt

a cut-down on the arm of a thrashing, hallucinating four-year-old. It took me almost an hour to do a procedure that on an adult would be accomplished in about ten minutes.

It was decided to treat Donna's burns with silver nitrate solution. It has the disadvantage of producing a permanent black stain on everything it touches — bed covers, floors, walls, uniforms — but it is one of the most effective antibacterial agents. Gauze was soaked in the silver nitrate solution and several layers were placed around Donna's legs. These dressings would have to be kept continuously saturated and changed every twelve hours. Twice a day I would examine the wounds and snip away any dead tissue.

The first forty-eight hours is the critical period in a burn case. Infection must be avoided; significant amounts of intravenous fluids should be delivered and urinary output kept at an adequate level. By the third day, maximum swelling is reached. Shortly after this, the patient goes into the diuresis phase, when the accumulated burn fluids are mobilized and excreted in the urine.

Following that, the next period is long and drawn out. It's called waiting. Waiting for the dead skin to come off. Waiting for the general health of the patient to improve. Waiting to make sure there are no complications. Then, perhaps two and a half or three weeks after the burn, when the patient has survived the life-threatening aspects of the acute injury, restoration can begin.

Donna had a couple of things going for her. Although the burns extended upward from her ankles, they did not cross the backs of the knees. I was fairly certain that she would avoid contraction of those joints and not be permanently crippled. I was also pretty sure that the necessary skin grafting could be accomplished in one operation. Large pieces of skin would be taken from her upper thighs and trimmed to fit the surface of the burn wounds. But we would wait until those wounds granulated — until tissue containing newly formed blood vessels appeared — for a granulated wound is an excellent bed for a skin graft. Still in all, young Donna was facing anywhere from eight to twelve weeks of hospitalization.

I hoped to God the Hancock family had medical insurance. The costs would be astronomical. Riddle of the day: how can a wiener roast turn into a holocaust?

I was still depressed when I got home, but Patsy had invited Boyd Falmouth, the senior surgery resident, and his wife Maryanne to join us for dessert and coffee. I liked Boyd, and since the Falmouths lived only a mile or so away, our two wives had become close. By the time they arrived, my spirits had revived, and we discussed politics, economics, the merits of the Dodgers, and the world situation in general. But, as usual, sooner or later, our talk turned to the hospital.

"The nurses on four were in absolute hysterics last night," Boyd said. "One of the patients was given the usual bottle of pHisoHex for his presurgical shower. About half an hour later, he pads out to the station in his robe and slippers and slams the empty bottle on the desk. 'Well,' he says, 'I'm nice and clean — and I also drank that damned stuff. God, it's horrible. The least they could do is flavor it with mint, or something.' " Laughing made Boyd sink back in his chair. "None of the nurses had the guts to tell him he was supposed to wash with the pHisoHex, not drink it."

Patsy got up to replenish the coffee. "Was he okay?" she asked.

"Sure," I said. "It's just a soap that fights bacteria. Nothing in it that would really hurt him."

"Unless you count diarrhea," Boyd laughed. "He got that — but good. And you should have heard him when the nurse came in to give him the presurgical enema."

I grinned. "That reminds me of a story I heard when I was an intern. Seems this high-powered, ulcer-prone executive was having trouble sleeping, so his family medic prescribed Nembutal rectal suppositories. A week later, the patient visited the office. 'How are you sleeping?' he was asked. 'Lousy,' was the reply. 'Look, doc, those big pills are hellishly hard to get down, but I swallow one every night, but for all the good they do, you can stick 'em up your ass!' "

"The party's getting rough," Maryanne chided.

Patsy nodded solemnly. "*Gross,* in fact."

"Speaking of gross," Boyd continued, "Don, have you ever operated with Dr. Warner?" I shook my head. "God, he drives me up the wall. He's a real butcher. Anyway, I guess this morning I wasn't moving fast enough for him. All of a sudden, he shouted, 'Don't fondle the tissue, Falmouth; I haven't got all day. If you want to fondle tissue, do it on weekends.' " Boyd grimaced. "Another thing about him that drives me crazy. He calls everybody 'cousin.' And he's got this habit of referring to the patient's tissue as 'meat' and the coagulator as the 'buzzer.' He spends half the time while he's operating saying, 'Buzz the meat, buzz the meat' — or 'Buzz, cuz . . . buzz, cuz.' One of these days I'm going to deck him."

I was about to remind Boyd that I didn't think that course of action too advisable, when the phone rang. I picked it up. It was the Administration Office at the hospital.

Word had just been received that a commercial jet, loaded with passengers, had crashed at the airport. Advance reports were still spotty, but all medical centers in the area had been placed on alert and were dispatching emergency vehicles to the scene. Available doctors were asked to report and stand by to treat the injured. I knew this was standard procedure in the case of major disasters. Even though there was a large municipal hospital located only a few miles from the airport, all of the injured would not be taken there. To avoid overloading any one facility, victims would be transported to several hospitals in the area.

"Dr. Falmouth is here with me," I said hurriedly into the phone. "We're on our way."

I handed Boyd his coat and slipped into my jacket. "No telling how long we'll be," Dr. Falmouth said to his wife, "so you'd better not wait for me to get back. When you're ready to leave, take the car. Don can drop me off at home when we're through."

As soon as we reached the hospital, we reported to Administration and the Emergency Room. No activity yet, so we headed for the doctors' lounge to wait. More than twenty physicians of every specialty, all hurriedly summoned like ourselves, sat wordlessly watching the television screen.

Mobile camera crews and news helicopters were already at the airport en masse. The broadcaster was asking sightseers to stay away from the area so that rescue operations would not be hampered, but at the same time, was going into great detail about which roads in the area were still open to traffic. Even as he spoke, hordes of curious onlookers in the background, realizing they might be on TV, waved at the camera.

There followed a picture of the carnage. A dense fog from the ocean had rolled in and visibility was poor. Evidently the plane had overshot the strip, crashed, and disintegrated. The fog imparted an eerie, unreal atmosphere, but there were bodies — or pieces of bodies — everywhere. No words could fully describe it.

Finally, the casualty count was announced. Out of the seventy-eight persons on the plane, seventy-seven were dead. The one survivor had eighty-five percent third-degree burns over his body. Every doctor in the lounge knew that he wouldn't last forty-eight hours. The television camera panned along the line of emergency vehicles from the surrounding communities.

None would be needed. The only function of the physicians who had accompanied the ambulances was to pronounce the dead, dead.

The television station, determined to milk the disaster, had sent a "man on the street" interviewer to talk to eyewitnesses. I have never been able to understand the morbid curiosity that disasters generate. Perhaps it is because people do not have an intimate encounter with death very often, and are fascinated by a preview of their own ultimate end.

Doctors are different, I suppose. We see so much death. Life and well-being are so damned precious to us. I was suddenly struck by the Herculean efforts we expend to save even one life. The surgeon who sweats six or eight hours to prevent death, or to repair or to reconstruct, is only the visible tip of a metaphorical iceberg made up of hundreds of teachers, researchers, technicians, nurses, administrators, and a vast armamentarium of equipment. I thought of the elation we experience when we save a single patient — and our outrage and frustration when we fail. We habitually recruited an army to save just one life — yet the loss of seventy-seven was turning into a circus.

As we watched the television screen, the interviewer stepped up to a young man eating a hamburger.

"I understand, sir," the broadcaster said, "that you were one of the first on the scene?"

"You bet," the youth mumbled between bites. "I got off work an hour or so ago, you know? And I was

driving home past the airport — and all of a sudden —
boom! Man, I mean — boom!!"

One of the doctors in the lounge got up and flicked
off the set. Boyd turned to me.

"Let's go. I feel a little sick."

Chapter Seven

THREE MONTHS HAD PASSED since I'd begun my plastic surgery residency. The first week remained vivid, and the ones that followed were equally hectic and challenging. Rounds, surgery, the clinic, conferences, and night calls — basically the routine was pretty much the same. There were follow-ups, of course, but mostly the patients changed like repertory actors in a perpetual drama.

I did the skin graft on the legs of Donna Hancock, our young burn victim. Many people think that after grafting, the patient's problems are over, but it's not true. Often, as months pass, grafted skin contracts and becomes wrinkled and irregular. Luckily for Donna, good progress has been made in dealing with this. Even skin that has healed by itself, without grafting, can form heavy, raised, ugly scars, but patients can now be fitted with support garments that lessen the amount of unsightly burn scar tissue. They are custom-made to fit any area of the patient's body and are similar to elastic support hose. The idea is to create pressure over the burned and grafted skin during healing, thereby keeping the tissue flat. I made arrangements for Donna to be fitted, but I knew that this therapy, although effective, is especially hard on kids. The support garments are uncomfortable and constrictive, and they have to be worn for at least six months. Once out of the hospital, Donna would have to come back every few weeks to be refitted, for the supports have a tendency to become loose. I also referred Mrs. Hancock to our Psychological Department to discuss the need for counseling to help with any emotional trauma her daughter might suffer as a result of the injury and treatments. All things considered, though, I think Donna is going to come through okay.

I also had seen Mrs. Baynes, our siliconosis patient, several times. As I'd suspected, the condition of her breasts was too catastrophic to respond to antibiotics or wet dressings. The solution would have to be a simple mastectomy of both breasts, but I wanted to give her the benefit of every outside chance. I didn't push, but finally she had agreed to the surgery. I remember the morning I first changed her dressing. As she gazed down at her flatness, and at the incisions on either side of her chest where her breasts had been, I expected an emotional reaction, but she was suprisingly calm.

"It's ugly — so ugly," she whispered.

I replaced the dressing and took her hand. "We were

extremely careful during the surgery, Mrs. Baynes," I said. "There's enough skin left for implants later — if you want them."

I could only guess the torment she was experiencing — this woman whose original fear of surgery had guided her to Mexico and the damned silicone injections.

"I'll let you know," she said quietly.

As long as we're on the subject of follow-ups, I guess everyone likes a success story. Betty Pearce, whose breast augmentation I had done during the first week of my residency, appeared one day at the clinic for her final checkup. She was wearing slacks and a cardigan sweater buttoned up the front, but her new silhouette told me I'd done my job well. Her husband was with her, ebullient as ever.

"Boy," Betty sighed with a smile, "am I beat! We just came from the Egyptian exhibit at the museum." She began unbuttoning her sweater; it was warm in the clinic. Her husband suddenly slipped the garment from her shoulders and grinned.

"Show him, honey!"

She was wearing a T-shirt with a reproduction of the King Tut mask over each breast. Emblazoned underneath were letters four inches high: *Don't touch my Tuts!*"

"He bought it for me this morning," Betty said, "and nothing would do but I wear it right away."

We all had a good laugh, and I thought I even detected the hint of a smile on Miss Farrell's face.

Colonel Bainbridge was still with us, but he was not doing well at all. Besides the large ulcer under his ear where the tumor had broken through the skin, a growth had developed on the left side of his neck, and another had appeared in front, over his windpipe. His pain was constant now, requiring ever larger doses of narcotics, but he bore his extreme discomfort with stoicism. I had become very fond of the elderly gentleman, and besides seeing him on rounds, I'd gotten into the habit of looking in on him whenever I could. I felt so sorry for his wife, too. The colonel had been moved from the Intensive Care Unit to a semi-private room and visiting hours were strict. When she couldn't be by his side, I was likely to find Mrs. Bainbridge in the visitors' lounge, sitting quietly, anxious not to be in the way. There was no way she could help. She knew it as well as anyone, but she got comfort from just being near her husband.

Some time before, Dr. Parmenter had started the colonel on anticancer drugs, and soon afterward decided to try injecting the medication directly into the arteries of the neck, hoping that it might bring the patient some relief from the excruciating pain. But neither of us had much hope that it would have any effect. We continued to search for any treatment that might help, knowing all the time that there was little that could be done. Colonel Bainbridge was a terminal case.

Over the weeks, in many brief talks with Mrs. Bainbridge, I'd always tried to adopt a positive, cheerful attitude, without actually lying. I don't know whom I was protecting, her or me. Spying her this morning, however, I decided the time had come to be a little more realistic. I gently explained that, in my opinion, her husband was beyond help and was going steadily downhill. She took it fairly well, as if she'd been expecting it all along. Most people have more grit than physicians suspect.

I think one of the most difficult tasks in medicine is to face the fact that your attempts at therapy have not been successful, to admit that the patient is going to die. It's like a personal battle lost.

I hated to leave Mrs. Bainbridge, but I was due in surgery. The first operation of the day was a reduction mammoplasty on Elsa Morehouse. I guess a lot of flat-chested women might find it difficult to understand why any woman would want such an operation — the removal of tissue to decrease the size of breasts. Mrs. Morehouse was a classic case. I'd first met her at the clinic, and I remembered our conversation.

"When I was a teenager," Mrs. Morehouse had confessed, "I thought I was pretty hot stuff. Sure, I enjoyed the wolf whistles from the boys." She'd shaken her head. "But my breasts kept getting bigger and bigger. Pretty soon, I was having trouble buying clothes. It seemed like I spent my life in tent dresses. When I dared to wear a bathing suit, I had to go to a special shop that sold two-piece suits separately. A size twelve bottom, and a forty-four top. I even tried a diet. I slimmed down everywhere else, but no matter how much weight I lost, my breast size seemed to stay the same."

I'd nodded. "It's known as macromastia, Mrs. Morehouse. Occasionally obesity compounds the condition, but nobody really knows what causes it. Some think it starts during puberty as a hormonal problem. Others just settle for heredity."

"By the time I got married," she'd continued, "I was wearing a size forty-four bra, with an E cup, and I'm only five feet four. I had four kids, and nursed them all. Maybe that had something to do with it, but as I got older, my breasts began to droop and they seemed heavier than ever. Lord, doctor, my back aches all the time." She'd let her fingers run over the deep grooves on her shoulders, where there were heavy calluses caused by pressure from her bra straps. "Then I heard about this operation. . . ." Her voice trailed off.

I'd checked her records. Forty-nine years old, an apparently happily married housewife, her family complete. The last fact was important because reduction mammoplasty is one cosmetic breast operation that does preclude future breast-feeding. Mrs. Morehouse had no history of cardiac or pulmonary diseases, which would make an operation under general anesthesia more perilous. There was no reason why she shouldn't have the requested surgery.

Before she'd left the clinic, we'd scheduled the operation. Dr. Parmenter and I would be doing it this morning.

The preoperative calculations, measurements, and

markings involved in a reduction mammoplasty are somewhat similar to what a designer goes through when planning a dress: we use a plastic pattern. With standards that have been worked out by surgeons, we decide on the new location for the nipple and the amount of skin and tissue to be removed.

In the operating room, we carefully traced the pattern on both breasts. Once the patient was asleep, we were ready to go. Dr. Parmenter did the right breast and I repeated the procedure on the left side.

Four and a half pounds of tissue were removed. When we'd finished, Mrs. Morehouse had moderate-sized breasts — molehills compared to the cumbersome mountains she had borne so long.

Our next scheduled operation was a facial dermabrasion, skin sandpapering. The patient was Thomas Gorleigh, an eighteen-year-old youth suffering the scarring aftereffects of acne. He'd be entering college soon and he wanted to put his best face forward.

Dr. Parmenter and I were in the middle of scrubbing, and Tommy was being wheeled upstairs, when the Surgical Supervisor advised us that our operating room had been preempted. A general surgeon had an emergency patient suffering acute internal injuries from an automobile accident. Dr. Parmenter sighed good-naturedly and nodded. This had happened several times since I'd been on his service. A patient with life-threatening injuries must be taken care of immediately. There wasn't a surgeon at University Hospital who hadn't encountered delays for the same reason. Plastic surgery cases, however, seemed a prime target when "bumping" was necessary, since most of our operations are elective and the necessary postponement involves no threat to the patient's well-being. It is annoying, nevertheless, to have your entire day's schedule thrown out of kilter. Many plastic surgeons, specializing in cosmetic cases and having the required volume, were opening small private hospitals to accommodate their patients and to circumvent this type of inconvenience.

Parmenter noticed my frown of frustration and smiled. "Don't fret it. You can't fight windmills." He was right. Eventually I'd learn to wage my battles only when there was a chance of winning.

"Don," Parmenter went on, "as long as we're delayed, I think I'll sit in on that staff meeting. Maybe you could do the workup and physical on Mrs. Quinn. Room 706. She checked in this morning for a tummy-tuck. But she's also complaining about her right wrist. Her family doctor thought it might be carpal-tunnel syndrome — but he admitted he's no expert. Take a look, will you?"

I nodded and headed for the room. After taking the medical history and doing a general physical, I turned my attention to Mrs. Quinn's wrist. Carpal-tunnel syndrome manifests some pretty clearcut symptoms. There is usually numbness of the thumb, the index and middle fingers, a weakness of grip, and intense burning pain. There was no doubt Mrs. Quinn's wrist

138

was painful, but the symptoms didn't match. I had just ordered X-rays when Parmenter phoned.

"I'm still in this meeting, but the operating room opened up. I didn't know how long you'd be tied up with Mrs. Quinn, so I told our number two man to go ahead on the dermabrasion with What's-His-Name assisting." What's-His-Name would be Dr. David Richman. As I've mentioned before, a different general surgery resident was assigned to our department on an eight-week rotating basis. Dr. Bob Sutton had moved on, and his successors came and went like a blur. "If you want to scrub in," Parmenter continued, "maybe you can help."

"Will do," I said, and headed for the surgical suite.

Dermabrasion, surgical planing of the skin, involves removal of the epidermis and a portion of the superficial layer of the dermis. It is usually employed to remove acne scarring or pockmarks. While it is impossible to remove deep pits, there is often about a fifty percent improvement in the appearance of the skin. Actually, the principle boils down to sanding off the high points so the low ones appear less deep. Even with the limitations of the technique, the results are generally satisfactory.

The first known practice of dermabrasion dates back to about 1905, with cylindrical knives being used. Later, surgeons progressed to using dental burs. In 1935, wire brushes were introduced, but it wasn't until the early 1950s that the technique that is used today — abrasive cylinders run by an air-driven motor — was developed. It allows very fine and easily controlled planing.

After scrubbing, I entered the operating room and donned my gown, gloves, and a huge face shield, similar to those worn by welders. As the sandpaper roller crosses the face, a considerable amount of bleeding results, and it is not uncommon for blood to be sprayed in every direction. During a dermabrasion procedure, a nurse spends a lot of time wiping the surgeon's face shield with a damp towel to permit unobstructed vision. Because of the emotional trauma that the blood and whirring sound of the dermabrader would cause the patient, we preferred to do the operation under general anesthesia.

As I approached the table, it was evident that things were not going well. Burke was literally screaming at Dr. Richman, who, through inexperience, had caused what might be a major problem. While working on Tommy's forehead, Dave had held the dermabrader too long over the same spot and a small burn of the skin resulted, about four millimeters in diameter — but, small or not, it was significant. All of us knew that we were working on a patient with a minor problem who was concerned with a good cosmetic result. How did you justify or explain a disfiguring scar that was not there before? Poor Dave stood hunched and penitent, and for the first time since I'd begun my plastic surgery residency, Burke seemed genuinely glad to see me.

Along with everything else, they'd been having trouble with the dermabrader. The machine was not sanding down the skin efficiently, and with a sigh of disgust, Dr. Burke straightened.

"Hold it—just hold up on everything for a minute," he instructed the team at large.

Between the two of us, we checked every connection on the sander, as well as the pressure gauge of the nitrogen tank that supplies the power for running the instrument. We weren't mechanics, but nothing seemed amiss—yet the rollers still were not operating at peak effectiveness. There was no alternative but to struggle along.

Burke began the delicate, fine work around the patient's nostrils, and a really serious problem developed—the tube that was inserted in Tommy's mouth somehow became dislodged and worked its way out of the trachea. This was a full-fledged emergency. We now had a patient who was anesthetized and could not breathe on his own; yet we had lost the access to the lungs by which we could breathe for him. If the tube weren't put back within three minutes, serious brain damage would occur. It was a situation that lent credence to Murphy's Law, "If something can go wrong, it will." Again we stopped, waiting while the anesthesiologist removed the endotracheal tube, and put a mask over Tommy's face. We cringed a little as it came into contact with our sterile operating field, but there was no choice. After fully oxygenating him, the anesthesiologist hurriedly put in a new tube. Luckily, he was successful. An experience like that makes you want to finish a case as soon as possible, but the

damned unsolved technical problem with the dermabrader forced us to go more slowly than usual. When
the procedure was finally completed, all of us had
frayed nerves.

As soon as Dr. Burke left, I took another look at the
forehead burn. The third day after a dermabrasion, a
thick scab forms. Then about a week later, it falls off,
leaving the patient's face unusually pink for two or
three months until normal color comes back. We
couldn't really be sure until later, but the burn didn't
seem too deep. We'd have to tell Tommy about the
mishap and hope for the best.

"Christ," moaned Dave. "This is like something out
of a bad movie script. A perfectly healthy kid comes in
with a few pockmarks — and I burn him, and then he
nearly suffocates." He turned to the nurses who were
about to wheel the patient to the recovery room.
"Hold on to him. He'll probably fall off the gurney on
the way back."

Later, when Tommy came in for his checkup, we
sighed with relief. There was no scar.

I was scrubbing for our final surgical procedure —
an otoplasty that I would be doing with Dr. Parmenter — when Dr. Burke came up behind me. He
seemed self-conscious, and what he had to say did not
come easy.

"I — I wanted to thank you for your help in there,"
he mumbled.

At that moment, I decided our childish little an-
tagonisms should stop. I realized that my resentment of

his personality had contributed as much to the friction between us as his attitude toward me. I didn't mind matching wits with the other services, or even with the patients, but the energy expended in sparring with Burke was a waste. We were both on the same side.

I met his eyes directly and smiled. "You're a fine surgeon, Al, and I want to learn. I'm anxious to do everything I can to help."

He visibly warmed. "Good. With Dr. Parmenter out of town all next month, I'm sure we'll get to know each other better."

I hid my surprise, reluctant to display my ignorance of Parmenter's plans.

"Well, we may have to work our tails off while he's away, but we'll handle it," I said.

"It doesn't work like that," he said ruefully. "An eerie thing happens when Larry's on vacation. It's like there's some damned underground tapping out the news that he's gone. I can't explain it, but almost everybody who needs plastic surgery seems to wait till he gets back." As the implication of that sank in, Burke walked away.

It was time that something went right, and I didn't anticipate any problems with the bilateral otoplasty on Mabel Herring. An otoplasty is an operation to correct prominent ears — to put them back in a more normal position in relation to the side of the head. Generally this type of surgery is performed on children, usually at about the time their friends and classmates begin to tease them. Evidently this woman had survived her childhood, but at twenty-six, had decided that she'd borne her defect long enough.

The operation is simple and works quite well. Most of the time the basic problem is that the cartilage does not have the folds that are present in the normal ear. With an adult, an otoplasty is done under local anesthesia and entails removing an elliptical piece of skin from behind the ear and moving a rasp or file back and forth to weaken the cartilage enough so that it can be bent. The newly formed folds are held in place by stitches.

I had seen the patient earlier and had considered her to be an emotionally stable woman. When we entered the operating room, she was wide awake, apparently impervious to the heavy sedation she'd been given. Since an otoplasty is a relatively simple procedure, we were not overly concerned, but shortly after we'd started, Mrs. Herring confessed to a phobia — she had a fear of having her feet and hands covered.

As in any operation, sterile drapes had been arranged to cover Mrs. Herring's body, leaving only the surgical area exposed. She became increasingly agitated.

"Doctor," she gasped, "I can't stand it — I'm burning up. I — I feel like I'm going to faint!" We glanced down at the patient. She was beginning to perspire, her face had paled, and her manner of speech indicated a true shortness of breath. Parmenter looked at me and then at the nurse.

"Fold the drapes back from Mrs. Herring's feet, please," he instructed. The nurse complied, and we continued. Only a few minutes passed.

"You're going to have to uncover my hands," the claustrophobic woman gasped. "Please."

Dr. Parmenter frowned. If we agreed, it would leave her unsterile hands dangerously close to our surgical field.

"I think I'm going to throw up," Mrs. Herring groaned. That convinced us that we could adjust to the situation, and we quickly folded the sheet back from her hands. At this point she relaxed, and the rest of the operation went smoothly. You just never know.

"What's with Mrs. Quinn?" I asked, as we were outside removing our gowns. "It doesn't look like carpal-tunnel syndrome to me."

"I haven't got all the tests back, but I agree," Parmenter replied.

"I almost wish it had been," I said longingly.

Ever sensitive, Dr. Parmenter stared at me for a moment, his fingers drumming thoughtfully at his side. "You haven't seen much hand surgery since you've been with me, have you, Don?"

I shrugged. "The orthopods get the juicy cases," I admitted.

Parmenter thought for a moment. "Do you know Eric Munssen?"

I knew he was one of the top surgeons in University Hospital's Orthopedic Department. "I've heard of him, but we've never met."

"He's a neighbor of mine, and we play tennis every Saturday. Last week he was telling me that one of the Ortho residents was out with hepatitis, and they're running a bit shorthanded." He pondered for a while.

"Did you know that I'm leaving next month for Europe? Be gone about four or five weeks. It might be a little slow while I'm away. If I can manage it, would you be interested in dividing your time and assisting Dr. Munssen?"

"You bet I'd be interested!"

It was absolutely vital that during my two years of plastic surgery training I become proficient at doing hand surgery. On the surface, it didn't sound unreasonable, but such experience was surprisingly hard to come by. Good hand surgeons willing to teach were few and far between, and there were hordes of residents in that specialty.

"Well, I'll see if I can reach Eric tonight," Parmenter promised. "Maybe we can all have lunch together soon."

I was jubilant. Being a protégé of the popular Chief of Plastic Surgery had many advantages. Things were looking great — but the day wasn't over yet.

I finished rounds about six forty-five P.M. All I had left to do before going home was to stop in the lobby and check on tomorrow's scheduled admissions. And that was good, because almost five weeks before, Patsy had written in to secure tickets to a popular musical at the Shubert Theatre. Tonight was the night, and with an eight-thirty curtain, we'd make it in time.

While I was waiting for the elevator, a nurse came running down the corridor. A few minutes before, one of the hospital's switchboard operators had received an anonymous call that an explosive device had been planted in the building, timed to go off at seven-thirty. Even as the nurse went along warning other members of the staff, the loud speakers blared.

"Code thirty-three, please. Code thirty-three."

The voice over the paging system was calm and matter of fact, deliberately kept that way to avoid frightening the patients. But every employee of the hospital knew that it was a signal to institute emergency procedure. There were periodic drills for fire, earthquakes, and bomb scares, with each situation designated by a different code number. Code thirty-three meant a bomb scare. All patients were to be moved from the back of the building to the front, which was deemed structurally stronger.

A bomb scare is frightening at any time, but University Hospital spanned two city blocks and was eight stories high. On this particular night, almost all of its nine hundred and seventy beds were filled. Nine hundred sick people — many not ambulatory — all of them terribly frightened. Every department fought possible chaos. In the surgical suites, operations already underway had to be completed — completed by nervous doctors and nurses. Patients already sedated for operations and just waiting were shuttled to and fro, with nobody knowing quite what to do with them. As time passed, sedation would have to be repeated. In the Renal Department, there were people on dialysis machines who could not be moved. In the cardiac Intensive Care Unit, there were heart patients whose lives depended on their not being upset or moved at all. In obstetrics, babies wouldn't wait to be born — and in the nursery, preemies were in incubators that were necessary to their lives. Other infants were carried from their controlled temperature and environment, and nurses ran around wondering where to put them. Many patients were hooked up to wall suction and oxygen, and there weren't enough portable units to go around. The Virology Department, concerned with research and testing for contagious diseases, madly tried to secure brimming tubes and beakers to prevent possible contamination. In the Physical Therapy Department, patients had to be fished from hydrotherapy pools, dried, and rushed to safety.

Every doctor, nurse, intern, and orderly was pushing patients' beds from the back of the building to the front. It resembled a demolition derby. I joined in, wondering what Godlike intellect had decided that one part of the hospital might be safer than another. Patients were babbling questions and those in the know, anxious not to alarm them, were mysteriously evasive, only adding to the growing uneasiness.

Before long the corridors were clogged with beds. I began carrying patients, while nurses trailed behind with their IV stands, catheter bags, and what-have-you. Just to save space, if they were physically able, I sat them up — three and four to each of the mattresses that had been placed on the corridor floors.

The hospital Security Department had joined with the police in searching the building. While we were dashing around, holding our breaths and watching the clocks, an in-house guard discovered a brown paper-wrapped package next to a soft-drink machine. A policeman gingerly took the box and handed it to the bomb squad, which deactivated it in a specially armored vehicle. Rumors spread that the bundle had contained two sticks of dynamite and a timing device, but there was really no way of knowing. Not only do I not know if the bomb was for real, but I never heard if anyone was ever apprehended.

Anyway, we began the laborious task of getting the patients back into their rooms. Then the page began crackling the names of staff doctors, for every floor nurse needed orders covering sedation for upset patients.

When the dust settled, I paused for a moment and looked out the window from one of the rooms. The building was surrounded by police cars and fire department trucks. Television crews had chosen advantageous positions, and a circling news helicopter added to the general din. The area had been cordoned off, and since it was now after seven, adjoining streets were clogged with the curious as well as visitors trying to reach the hospital. There had obviously been a news bulletin about the bomb scare, for the hospital's switchboard was deluged.

It was well after eight before I could get an outside line to call Patsy, and I knew I would lose at least another hour working my way through the unbelievable traffic jam that had been created.

"I heard about it on the radio," my wife volunteered. "I didn't bother to get dressed, but I double-checked the tickets." There was a pause. "Row E, seats 127 and 128," she monotoned. There was a silence so long that I thought the distraught switchboard operator might have disconnected us.

"Patsy . . . are you still there?"

"Yes. I was just checking the fine print. It says, 'Positively no refunds or exchanges.' "

Chapter Eight

WELL, I WANTED EXPERIENCE in hand surgery, and I got it.

Before Dr. Parmenter left, he managed my introduction to Dr. Eric Munssen. Joining them for lunch, I was quick to realize that they had already worked out the arrangement. Any time I was available during the next month and Munssen had surgery scheduled, I would assist. With everything settled, I was able to enjoy our meeting, all the time gaining insight into Dr. Munssen's personality.

Dr. Munssen was about forty-seven years old. He'd been born in Malmö, Sweden. Tall, blond, ruddy-faced, a shade over six feet, and a lean hundred and seventy pounds, he more closely resembled a champion skier than a surgeon. What intrigued me most was his methodical and punctilious manner — the hallmark of many hand surgeons. Even in the relatively simple ritual of eating, there was a rhythm to his selection of food — a bite of poached salmon, a piece of tomato, a mouthful of lettuce, a sip of coffee — an unvarying pattern repeated with utter precision. I sensed that he was a finicky perfectionist, but he was soft-spoken and polite. No doubt about it — I was going to enjoy working with Dr. Eric Munssen.

Hand surgery is a complicated specialty. Restoration of function takes priority over appearance, but it is great if both can be accomplished. The man sitting opposite me was a master at it. We had almost finished eating when he turned to me with a smile.

"You know, Don," he said, "the unique anatomy of the human hand and its amazing capacity to function have shaped the world. The hand is synonymous with touching. The other senses — taste, hearing, sight, and smell — they're all more acute in animals. Touch is the only sense which is most highly developed in man. We who have elected to repair hands have a great responsibility." With Dr. Munssen's slight accent, the words, which might have sounded pompous from anyone else, took on a special charm and grace.

The first case we did together was an implant arthroplasty — a replacement of the knuckles of a patient suffering from rheumatoid arthritis.

Louise Bonney was a middle-aged widow who had been supporting herself by working as a waitress in a local restaurant. I talked to her the night before the surgery was scheduled.

"Waiting tables is all I know, Dr. Moynihan," she

whispered, "and I just can't do it any more." She glanced down at the gnarled and swollen fingers that imparted a clawlike appearance to her hands. "Every time I pick up a dish or a glass, it hurts so bad I can't stand it. I even have to get a busboy to open a catsup bottle or mustard jar. And Mr. Farrow — he's the manager — said that the way my hands look is offending the patrons." Tears were close.

I patted her shoulder sympathetically. Dr. Munssen had told me that when he'd first seen Mrs. Bonney, she'd been extremely depressed over her physical state and confided that she had contemplated suicide. He had little doubt that she was serious.

"Ten years ago, we couldn't have helped you much," I said. "Now we can."

She nodded, and I felt her eyes following me from the room.

The replacement of knuckles with silicone joint prostheses has gained widespread acceptance. It's an interesting and satisfying operation. Artificial knuckles have been available only about nine or ten years, but their impact on hand surgery has been significant. They provide good function in place of joints that are almost totally useless. They offer hope where there was no hope before.

Because of the technique used, operating on hands is different from most procedures — and is a surgeon's dream! He operates in a clean, bloodless field.

A pneumatic tourniquet, which resembles a blood-pressure cuff, is placed around the upper arm. Before the tourniquet is inflated, the entire area below the cuff is tightly wrapped with a rubber bandage, emptying the hand and arm of all blood. Then the tourniquet is tightened, preventing blood replacement. Thus, during the surgical procedure, there is absolutely no bleeding. The tourniquet can be left on for as long as ninety minutes. Most hand operations are performed under nerve-block anesthesia, with the patient heavily sedated.

My early appearance in the operating room showed my eagerness, and when Dr. Munssen came in, he greeted me with a smile.

"Ready?"

"Ready."

As soon as Mrs. Bonney's arm had been prepared and anesthetized, I watched as Dr. Munssen made a comparatively shallow incision about one centimeter below the knuckle ridge toward the wrist. Then, working together, we preserved and retracted the large veins leading from the fingers, the nerve branches, and the extensor tendons. Dr. Munssen was so enthusiastic about his work that he became a delightful verbal encyclopedia.

"You know," he ruminated, "many physicians still cling to the belief that surgery like this should be considered only as a last resort." He shook his head sadly. "The old-guard rheumatologists in particular have tended to 'protect' their patients from surgeons until advanced deformities have left no alternative. But little by little, they're coming around."

As he talked, Munssen excised the diseased joints and cored out the adjacent bones so that the artificial knuckles could be inserted and stabilized.

"It's extremely important to use prostheses that fit exactly." Munssen indicated to a nurse that he was ready for the test implants that are used to determine which of the eight sizes available is proper for each joint. He spent considerable time trying, fitting, testing, and rejecting before he nodded his approval.

Each of the silicone prostheses resembled a human knuckle with wedge-shaped appurtenances at the top and bottom. They are designed so the protruding ends can be inserted into the adjacent bones.

Once Munssen had inserted the artificial knuckles, he closed the skin and applied a soft bulky dressing and a plaster splint. After a week or ten days, when the sutures were removed, the patient would be fitted with a light metal splint, and active finger motion would be encouraged. Eight weeks after surgery, Mrs. Bonney's hand would probably have regained a good range of active, painless motion. In three months or so, the other hand would be operated on, and she could go on with her life.

I was still in the locker room when I received a call from the floor nurse that Colonel Bainbridge had just died. He'd been growing weaker and weaker, and the cancer had become so extensive and painful that he'd been unable to take food. Even swallowing liquids was a chore. I had seen him early that morning and he had been in a coma. For his sake, I'd found myself wishing that the end would come quickly. There was nothing left for him except pain and misery.

I think I have learned fairly well that a doctor, to keep his sanity, mustn't get emotionally involved with his patients. He must take death in his stride. Nevertheless, as I watched the colonel valiantly struggle against impossible odds for many weeks, I'd grown to admire him tremendously. I felt a great sense of personal loss.

I had to certify his death, so I headed for the room. Then I was faced with the unpleasant task of informing Mrs. Bainbridge. The lounge was empty; the nurses remarked that they hadn't seen the colonel's wife that morning. I didn't relish breaking unhappy news over the phone; still, it was better than having Mrs. Bainbridge arrive at the hospital unprepared. I called her house and gently broke the news. After a few moments of silence, she thanked me for informing her and expressed her gratitude for my help over the rough times. She volunteered that she would get to the hospital and make arrangements as soon as possible, but there might be a delay because she had transportation problems. As she explained, my stomach bumped a couple of times and turned over. Someone had rewarded this courageous woman on the morning of her husband's death by stealing her car!

I would guess that during the time I was working with Dr. Munssen, I scrubbed in on perhaps forty hand cases. Some were minor and some were routine, but one of the most interesting involved an eighteen-year-old by the name of Scotty Ihnen.

He'd been having a good time in a tavern when he'd slipped and fallen on his own beer bottle, sustaining a small but deep cut in the palm of his hand. Although he didn't know it at the time, the jagged glass had severed both tendons to the middle finger.

At University Hospital's Emergency Room, the doctor on duty examined the wound and realized that it was in the part of the hand called "no man's land." There is an anatomical sheath in this area that keeps the tendons in place. Any repair of lacerations within it often causes the tendons to adhere to each other. Therefore the E.R. doctor had only stitched up the skin and arranged an appointment for the patient with Dr. Munssen.

The surgery was scheduled and Mr. Ihnen was admitted. Tests were made and he was listed as the first surgical case the following morning. Accordingly, I stopped in to see him on evening rounds.

He assessed my mood. "Look, doc — how about letting me go home for the night, and I'll come back first thing in the morning?"

I stared at him, trying to decide if he was serious. He was. "No way," I said.

"Come on, Dr. Moynihan," he wheedled; "I got something to take care of."

"I'm sorry, but it's impossible. This is a hospital, not a hotel," I said firmly. "We have to know exactly what you eat and drink. There are certain medications ordered, and we want to be sure you get a good night's sleep. So forget it. I'll see you in the morning."

Later that night, Patsy and I were watching the nine o'clock news. Suddenly I inched forward on my chair and stared intently at the screen.

"Don?"

Without taking my eyes from the set, I held up a finger, stopping my wife in midsentence. We watched — I with delighted satisfaction; Patsy curiously. It was the typical on-camera human-interest vignette — a famous soccer player being plied with questions by a woman interviewer. When it was over, I leaned back with a sigh of gratification.

"I didn't know you were so fascinated with soccer," Patsy said.

I shook my head. "I'm not. But did you see the woman doing the interviewing?"

Patsy nodded. "She's new, I think. Attractive. Has a nice style."

The on-camera interviewer had been Kristina Healy, my face-lift patient of some months ago. I remembered her doubts and qualms. Now she looked a good ten years younger. She looked sensational, in fact. Her new appearance had moved her from behind the camera to in front of it. It was nice to know that I'd played a small part in a new and rewarding career.

While I was still glowing, the hospital called. Scotty Ihnen was missing. The nurse relayed what little they'd been able to reconstruct. Around seven, as the visitors began pouring in, someone had seen Scotty on his way to the lobby. Since he was in bathrobe and loafers, it was assumed that he was meeting a friend downstairs. He hadn't been missed until visiting hours were over and the staff had settled into its normal nighttime routine.

"He'll be back," I halfheartedly assured the nurse.

"What makes you think so?"

"Just a hunch," I said. I was reluctant to admit that I had been forewarned.

I was restless that night, and called the hospital several times to see if our patient had reappeared. He hadn't. By the time I arrived to make early rounds at six o'clock, his room was still empty.

I was muttering curses and expecting to see a deserted bed when I poked my head in at seven. Instead, Scotty was propped against the pillows, grinning a good morning. Unknowingly, he had timed his return just right — in the middle of the nursing shift change. No one had seen him sneak back. He had managed to materialize as mysteriously as he had disappeared.

"Of all the stupid stunts . . . ," I exploded.

"Cool it, doc," Scotty said. "I told you it was important. I'm here. So everything's okay — right?"

The operation was scheduled to begin in about an hour and the anesthesiologist, who was a real prima donna, wanted to cancel the procedure. What if the patient had eaten, or taken drugs, he argued? What difference did it make, I countered, we were doing the surgery under a nerve block. I hung in, and finally the anesthesiologist compromised. If I would repeat certain tests to make sure Scotty's vital signs hadn't changed, they would schedule a kidney operation first, and move Scotty down to the second procedure of the morning. I quickly agreed.

I needn't have worried about Dr. Munssen's reaction to the bizarre events of the previous night. He had gotten up that morning with the sniffles and a slight fever, and had asked Dr. Bruce Durham, who was Chief of Orthopedics, to do the case instead of him.

The Surgical Supervisor got in touch with Dr. Durham and advised him of the change of schedule. Following a little sweet talk from me, she merely told him that the surgical sequence had been rearranged and that the Ihnen operation was now set for ten A.M.

When the Fates start to frown, they do it with vengeance. The urology procedure, which should have taken two hours, stretched out to four. A kidney stone that couldn't be passed and an extremely slow surgeon accounted for the delay. So there I was, sitting with the powerful Chief of Orthopedics, both of us twiddling our thumbs and trying to make small talk for two hours, when we were supposed to be operating. We were waiting in an office outside the operating room, and every five or ten minutes, I dashed to the surgical suite to see how things were going. Slowly — that's how things were going. The Chief of Orthopedic Surgery was becoming progressively more irritable at the waste of his valuable time. He finally apologized for his foul humor. It wasn't only the delayed surgery, he confided, but several of his orthopedic residents had been complaining that some goddamned son-of-a-bitch from another service was screwing them out of some juicy teaching cases. Dr. Durham didn't know that the "goddamned son-of-a-bitch" was sitting about ten feet away from him. Feeling as if I were perched on the edge of a volcano, I spent the rest of the time trying to divert him from the subject. Finally, at five minutes before noon, we began the Ihnen surgery.

I was glad when it was over. Dr. Durham turned out to be a complete spastic in the operating room. I found out later that he was known among the other residents as "Super-Twitch." Extremely nervous, he was constantly bouncing up and down, stamping his feet, shaking his head, moaning, and groaning. His shenanigans made it almost impossible to concentrate on the procedure.

Scotty did well after the surgery. He had to be kept in a cast for about three weeks so the tendon could heal. The time came when he reported to the Outpatient Clinic and I removed the stitches and applied a lighter splint. As it turned out, that was the last time I ever saw him. I knew that he would botch up the results of his operation if he weren't under proper medical care, and I spent hours trying to locate him by phone, but he had disappeared. I could only guess that he'd taken the splint off himself. It bothered me that I would never know if the end result of the surgery was a success or a failure.

It was just as well that Dr. Munssen decided to nurse his cold for another day and postpone his surgical cases.

The Harrises were back with their baby son George, and Dr. Burke had scheduled the removal of the giant hairy nevus from the child's shoulder and arm. I would be assisting, and in view of our previous encounters with the parents, neither of us was looking forward to the experience.

Burke had wangled an eight A.M. starting time, hoping to give Mrs. Harris as little time as possible in which to become hysterical, but we didn't get going until well past nine. One reason for the delay was that the operating room was too cool. The heat loss in infants during surgery is greater than with adults, and the anesthesiologist insisted that the room temperature be above seventy-two degrees. No one, however, had thought to tell the engineer whose job it was to oversee the temperature controls, and he had disappeared for coffee. It seemed that we were faced with a strong union situation, and nobody but the engineer dared change the controls. So there was nothing to do but wait until he returned — and then wait some more for the temperature to rise to the desired level.

The floor nurse had explained the delay to Mrs. Harris but couldn't seem to get through to her. We got the report that the child's mother was distraught, smothering her small son with hugs and kisses as though she would never see him again.

While we were sitting and waiting for the O.R. thermometer to creep up, Burke looked at me morosely.

"What would you think about doing the whole procedure this morning?" he asked. The birthmark was large and, to reduce the trauma, we had planned to remove the growth in several operations at widely spaced intervals.

I hesitated. "It's a lot of surgery for a little kid."

"I know," Burke said. "But if we stretch this out, Mrs. Harris is going to end up on the funny farm — or she's going to turn Georgie into the world's youngest psycho. The boy's in good shape, and I don't foresee any problems."

There was truth in what he said, and I nodded.

So we completely removed the birthmark. We incised around the entire circumference of the growth and removed all of the hairy, abnormal skin. Then we took a split-thickness skin graft from the child's back and placed it over the wound. Everything went remarkably well.

George's mother was waiting for us immediately outside the operating room door. Sobbing and nearly hysterical, she followed the child all the way to the recovery room and, when barred from entering, pulled a chair up to the door and sat there for the next two hours. Once George was back on the pediatrics ward, all hell broke loose. Mrs. Harris had Dr. Burke paged regularly every hour with some imagined crisis. Perhaps he was suffering guilt pangs for his aggressive handling of the birthmark; at any rate, Burke sprinted to the room at each summons. But George was doing fine. Finally, late in the afternoon, when another call came, Burke confessed he'd had it.

"Don, it's getting hard for me to be civil to Mrs. Harris. I know she's concerned, but she's got my teeth on edge. I'd say she's got an IQ about equal to her son's age." He squared his shoulders. "Maybe that's the answer. Remember Miss Farrell's approach and how well it worked? Mrs. Harris may be a mother, but she's also a spoiled, pampered brat. I'm going to tell her that if she cries wolf once more, I am going to see that she and her husband are thrown out of the hospital."

Burke's tactics worked like a charm. Thereafter, Georgie's convalescence proceeded without further incident.

Once every week there was a senior staff luncheon, and when Gloria Velasquez appeared at the Emergency Room, Dr. Munssen was at the meeting, so I took the call instead. The seventeen-year-old Mexican girl who sat watching the E.R. doctor clean up her hand looked like a Madonna. Her liquid brown eyes were pools of reflected innocence, and her fragility made everyone especially gentle and solicitous. I took down the details of the injury, beginning with the standard question.

"How did it happen?"

"A cut — with a knife."

"Accident?"

"I wouldn't exactly say that." A hint of a sardonic smile accompanied her answer, and I suddenly sensed cold steel under her angelic demeanor.

With a little perseverance, I got the story. Another

girl had tried to stab her in the neck with a switch-blade. In an attempt to protect herself, Gloria had grabbed the blade, suffering several superficial cuts on her palm and a much deeper slash across her little finger. Looking at it, I had no doubt that the tendons had been severed. But her quick reaction probably saved her life.

"Did the police bring you in?" I asked. She shook her head. "Are you going to report the assault?"

"No. And there's no sense of your doing it. I'll deny it." She met my gaze defiantly. "Officer, I was slicing this loaf of bread . . . ," she rehearsed in a monotone.

I shrugged. "What happened to the other girl — the one who attacked you?"

Her lips parted in a satisfied smile. "I kicked the shit out of her!"

We kept talking and, little by little, Gloria's past unfolded. It was quite a story. If there was any kind of trouble she hadn't gotten into, it was only because she hadn't gotten around to it. The reason for the knife attack was that Gloria had grabbed the other girl's boy-friend. Our patient did not attend school; she'd been thrown out a number of times. She didn't work, either. Her parents had disappeared — maybe gone back to Mexico. She admitted that she smoked a lot of mari-juana, and enjoyed hard drugs when she could get them. I could only guess how she occupied her time and got enough money for her pleasures. She showed me the picture of her two-year-old daughter. She'd had the child when she was fifteen.

By now Dr. Munssen was available and we conferred. With the patient's unstable history, we decided to admit her immediately. Gloria was like a beautiful, wary animal, mapping escape routes if needed, glancing with distrust at everyone who approached her. Once she left, we'd probably never see her again.

The operation proved interesting. Although the skin wound itself was in no-man's-land, Gloria's action of closing her hand about the knife had caused her fingers to be flexed when the slashing occurred. The tendon, instead of being severed in the region where it should not be repaired, had been stretched beyond that critical area. There was enough length so that it could be pulled up and stitched at the end of the finger.

Before she was discharged, I had another chat with her.

"You're going to have to keep that cast on for a while," I cautioned her. "Will you be able to get along?"

"Sure."

"What about taking care of your baby?"

"Some friends keep her for me."

"I want you to come back and see me at the clinic in one week."

"Okay."

"Promise?"

She crossed herself. "I swear it — on the memory of my mother."

True to her word, Gloria appeared as scheduled. Her cast was completely covered with signatures, cartoons, and doodles — mementos from all her friends. She pointed at a prominently scrawled name.

"That's her." She met my baffled eyes. "The girl who stabbed me." It was obvious that the barrio had a code of its own.

Gloria was doing just fine, but we decided that the cast should stay on another ten days or so. I told her the date I would expect her back.

"Sorry, doc," she said loftily, "I'm leaving for Colorado tomorrow."

"Why Colorado?"

"Why not? Tomorrow, Colorado — next stop, the moon," she grinned.

"When will you be back?"

"I won't be coming back."

It was much too early to remove the sutures and the cast to evaluate the finger's ability to flex. To say that I was disgruntled was putting it mildly. All my arguments were useless. A compromise was in order.

"If I get you a transcript of your records, will you promise to go to a clinic in Colorado?"

She thought about it. "Maybe."

Poor Gloria. For all her faults, she had a special sense of honor. She did not make promises that she wasn't sure she'd keep. I was depressed after she left, and the fact that I would never know the results of my surgery was only part of it. Kids like Gloria had so much against them. I hoped that she would find a better life — or whatever it was she was searching for. I could repair a hand, but there was nothing I could do to fix her other problems.

Chapter Nine

M Y STINT WITH DR. MUNSSEN had come to an end. Dr. Parmenter got back, and for six weeks we worked ourselves into the ground. As Burke had warned, it had been slow while the boss had been away, but suddenly it seemed that everyone in the area who had cosmetic or reconstructive problems began filing in and demanding appointments. Many were anxious to have their surgery before the Thanksgiving and Yuletide holidays. I wasn't getting enough sleep, and I spent a great proportion of my off-call weekend time in bed, trying to catch up. One of the things that sustained me was the fact that Patsy and I would be going to the big plastic surgery convention scheduled for mid-November in Miami, Florida.

When major conventions in any specialty were held, it was policy for two of the staff doctors in that particular field to attend, with University Hospital picking up the tab. Dr. and Mrs. Parmenter would be going, of course, and Dr. Burke had been given the option of either attending the upcoming meeting or going to a May convention that was to convene in Honolulu. After a family conference, Dr. Burke had decided that Hawaii was more to his taste; therefore, the invitation to the Miami gathering was extended to me. Patsy was already haunting the maternity shops assembling a suitable wardrobe.

In the blur of cases that marked the period before we left, several stand out.

I received a phone call early one morning from Mrs. Baynes. Now that the bilateral mastectomy that had removed her silicone-rotted breasts had healed, she'd decided to undergo implant surgery. I was delighted. We'd become good friends, and she'd told me that every time she looked at her flat chest, rightly or wrongly it reminded her of her stupidity. Even during the phone call I sensed her hesitation at the big decision for additional surgery, and I hastened to assure her that, in my opinion, she was doing the right thing. She agreed to being admitted the next day, before she could change her mind, and I told her I'd make sure she'd be on the same floor as before, where she'd know the nurses and see familiar faces.

In earlier talks, I had explained that the breast implants would have a slightly different contour from the real things, but they would provide the shape she wanted. I had also explained that we could, at a later date, reconstruct areola areas — the darker skin around the nipples — and nipples themselves. But she hadn't seemed too interested. At any rate, the implantation surgery went without a hitch, and when we finished, she had a very acceptable figure.

And then there was Paula Florendez. She had undergone augmentation mammoplasty in a Brazilian city where she'd lived; then her husband had been transferred to California. In the meantime, a problem had developed with the implant in her left breast. A tight tissue capsule had formed, which made the breast too firm and gave it an irregular appearance. We'd decided that the best course of action was to remove the capsule and reposition the prosthesis. She was admitted to the hospital, and it didn't take long to discover that Mrs. Florendez was a difficult patient. Every time I entered the room, she and her husband were engaged in a non-stop argument. It was apparent that they were having serious marital problems.

On one occasion, after her husband had stormed from the room in a huff, Mrs. Florendez confided that her mate had started to play around shortly after their wedding. One of the reasons she had decided to have augmentation mammoplasty in the first place was to increase her appeal to him.

Had we not been so rushed when we saw her originally, we might have been more wary before agreeing to the corrective surgery. Mrs. Florendez had made several appointments for the operation and then canceled them at the last moment — one time using the excuse that the specified date was her birthday. Later, when we took down her history, we noticed that her birthday was still three months in the future.

She had also told us that during her last surgery, she'd had a severe reaction to the general anesthetic that had been utilized, but she was completely vague about what drugs or techniques had been used. When questioned for details, she couldn't remember. We could only guess that she was allergic to halothane, a widely used gas — but we couldn't be sure. Unwilling to take chances, Parmenter decided to do the corrective surgery under local anesthesia.

By the time we'd gotten halfway through the operation, the Chief of Plastic Surgery not only regretted that decision, but I suspect he would have been deliriously happy if he'd never laid eyes on Mrs. Florendez. Our patient began to scream at the first needle and continued her hysterics throughout the entire operation. Between our placating her and employing all sorts of desperate gambits to ease her tension, the surgery took over two hours. Had it been done under a general anesthetic, it would easily have been completed in half that time. Nevertheless, we struggled doggedly, eventually getting the capsule out and the implant back into a satisfactory position. Both Dr. Parmenter and I breathed a sigh of relief when the dressing was on and Mrs. Florendez was wheeled from the operating room.

However, our troubles with this one weren't over yet. About four hours after the surgery, she and her husband came storming into my office.

"I'm going home," Mrs. Florendez announced. "I'm getting out of this crummy hospital right now!"

She had a dozen fabricated reasons. The hospital was no good, the nurses were incompetent, an intern had insulted her, the food was fit only for pigs, the television reception was lousy, and the woman with whom she was sharing a room was a pain in the ass.

I kept her talking, and from one or two comments she made, it finally dawned on me that the actual reason why she was insisting on being discharged was panic. She had no intention of leaving her husband alone for the normal two days of hospitalization because she suspected that he would be cheating on her.

I argued for a while, but finally shrugged. Any patient can leave a hospital whenever he or she desires. It is policy to reason with him and point out the consequences, but in the end, there is no way to prevent his leaving. And after encountering two or three such cases, the wise doctor finds himself wondering if, all things considered, he wants them to stay. Experience has proven that these are very difficult patients, whose disruptive personalities can spell real trouble for the entire staff. I pointed out to Mrs. Florendez that if she were to leave, it would be necessary that she sign an "Against Medical Advice" release form, relieving the hospital and the physicians of any responsibility for the consequences of her action. She quickly agreed.

The second case, a rhinoplasty, was memorable for several reasons. I had seen the patient — Celeste Bigliani — on the very first day of my plastic surgery residency. When months passed without her calling for an appointment, I had thought that her mother, who had been so opposed to the surgery, had won out. Actually, Celeste had been waiting for her annual vacation.

Also, it was the first female nose job I did completely on my own. I had assisted on quite a few rhinoplasties on women, and had acted as primary surgeon on any number of males, who generally had broken noses from fights or injuries of one sort or another. The main difference was that the men had not been particularly interested in attaining esthetically perfect contours; they just wanted their noses straightened and functional again.

But Celeste Bigliani was a beautiful girl, and since she had been my very first patient on this service, I felt a proprietary interest.

Although Dr. Parmenter had scrubbed with me, just before we were ready to start he confessed to feeling a bit feverish and nauseated — the flu bug was rampant. Rather than cancel, he suggested that I go ahead with our current rotating assistant. It surprised me how far I had come in six months, how the constant surgery had built my confidence and refined my expertise. I felt no qualms.

Emotionally, Miss Bigliani was an ideal patient. She wanted her surgery more than almost anything in the world. The operation was completed without incident, and the nose was taped and splinted in its new form. I had a hunch that the results would satisfy even my desire for near perfection.

The day after the surgery, I entered Miss Bigliani's room and found her quietly crying, carefully muffling the sobs. She was doing well, so I was momentarily baffled. She caught my eye and gestured that I should draw the curtains that afforded privacy.

"I feel awful," she confessed softly.

I instinctively reached out to take her pulse, but she drew her wrist away.

"I'm all right. But Linda . . . the girl in the next bed?" I nodded for her to go on. The patient sharing the room was not one of mine, but I'd casually noticed her when I'd come in. An absolutely lovely blonde of about nineteen, she had smiled a warm but silent greeting.

"She has bone cancer!" Celeste's voice was an agonized whisper. "And she knows it's terminal. She *knows!*" The silent tears started again. "I feel so guilty. I mean, all this fuss about my nose — and there she is, dying!"

"I'm going to have your room changed, Celeste," I said firmly. My patient's eyes widened, and her self-recrimination became more intense.

"No! I couldn't do that. She'd know the reason. God, what would she think?"

Now I knew that even if I moved her, the image of the dying girl would remain. I took a different tack.

"At least you're company for her, so you're helping," I reasoned. "But if it gets too much for you, let me know, and we'll make a change." Celeste shook her head.

From that time on, I never again risked imposing added depression on my cosmetic surgery patients. Completely unfounded though it is, most of them feel a twinge of guilt at their supposed vanity, and they don't need unnecessary coals heaped on the fire. I had a memo to the Admitting Office prepared for Dr. Parmenter's signature, explaining the situation and requesting that, whenever possible, cosmetic surgery cases be paired with patients recovering from insignificant operations or minor injuries.

Soon after that, Patsy and I flew to Miami for the convention, leaving on a Sunday and arriving that night at the Miami resort hotel where the meeting would be held. Official registration was not scheduled until the next morning, but the premises were already swarming with plastic surgeons and their wives, and we were handed a thick guide to the activities that would be offered during the next five days.

It has been said that medical conventions are merely convenient tax-exempt vacations for doctors and their spouses. It's true that they are always held in a vacationers' paradise such as Las Vegas, San Francisco, or Nassau. The program always includes formal dinners and dances, which give everyone a chance to dress up. Oddly enough, the plastic surgeons often outshine their wives, strutting around like peacocks in gaudy, expensive clothes. More than in any other specialty, those in plastic surgery are concerned with appearance, image, and the impression of affluence. The lobby was like a constantly moving kaleidoscope. But an unbelievable amount of information, knowledge, and new techniques is offered at these conventions. And in addition to being given this opportunity for learning, we also had a chance to rub and polish our minds against the brains of others in the same field. Lectures, slides, movies, symposia, and actual operations live on television were scheduled every day from eight in the morning until seven at night. At all times, there were five or six simultaneous activities so that the surgeons could choose the subject that most interested them.

I thumbed through the program. There was a panel session discussing the newest techniques for treating midfacial fractures, a lecture on acid burns, a demonstration of laser surgery, a symposium concerned with the survival rates in mastectomies. All in all, over a hundred separate lectures on widely varied subjects were offered, plus a horde of technical and scientific exhibits. In no other way could such a vast amount of knowledge be gleaned in so short a time.

I pointed out a page to Patsy headed "Ladies' Activities." The Women's Hospitality Committee had been busy, determined that the wives would not be bored while their husbands were attending the scientific sessions. Patsy pounced on one particular notation.

"A plastic surgeons' art exhibit?" she asked. "What do you suppose that is?"

I grinned and tried to explain. Plastic surgeons are unique. They see themselves not only as scientists but also as artists. In their minds, they create beauty — just

176

as surely as any Rembrandt, Michelangelo, or Rodin
—and they're proud of it. But it is not enough that
they are convinced. There must be tangible evidence
of their talent and creativity to show the world. Many
plastic surgeons I knew had artistic hobbies: painting
in water colors or oils, making ceramics, doing wire or
clay or paper sculpture, wood carving, photography,
even glassblowing.

Once I was home from the activity-packed week,
there was a day's lull, which helped me over the inevitable jet lag, and then I drew a clinically interesting, but personally disturbing, case.

Twelve-year-old Walter Putnam was an honor student and the only son of upper-income parents who
lived in a home among the foothills that fringed the
city. Walt and a friend had been playing a Bonnie-and-
Clyde game with his father's supposedly unloaded
shotgun. The other boy had playfully pointed the gun
and threatened to shoot. Our patient had said, "Go
ahead," and, in response to the dare, the youth had
pulled the trigger. The blast had carried away a large
portion of Walt's chin and had left a gaping hole the
size of a silver dollar through his left shoulder from
front to back.

The victim had been rushed to a neighborhood hospital, where, fortunately, a very good general surgeon
was on call. Everyone agreed that Walt's guardian
angel had been on active duty; no major blood vessel
had been severed, although the charge had barely
missed the main artery in the shoulder. But the left

upper chest and jaw of what had once been an extremely handsome youngster now resembled raw meat.

The staff surgeon had immediately performed a tracheostomy to make sure that Walt would not suffocate if the injury caused breathing problems. He had cleaned and removed the dead tissue from the wounds, temporarily stitched the skin together where he could, packed the open areas of the shoulder and jaw with sterile gauze, ordered antibiotic soaks, and kept the patient under close observation in the I.C.U. for twelve hours. Then, facing the fact that his medical facility did not have a plastic surgery department, he requested the youth's transfer to University Hospital.

Dr. Parmenter, Dr. Burke, and I conferred on a step-by-step plan of treatment. It had taken a fraction of a second to inflict the wounds. With all the medical and scientific means at our command, it would take the three of us many months to repair the damage, and partial repair was all we could hope for. The perfectly handsome lad would never be perfect again.

Our strategy called for continuing the antibiotic-soaked packs for another two days to reduce the risk of infection, and scheduling the first of numerous surgical procedures for the following week.

In Walt's case, we originally thought that two skin flaps would be needed for padding — one for the shoulder and one for the jaw — but we were elated to discover that the shoulder injury seemed to be filling in and healing nicely. We adopted a wait-and-see attitude. As time passed, we were certain that a simple skin graft would effect the necessary closing of the wound. Although the shoulder would always have a concave indentation, the graft was by far the more desirable procedure.

So, during the initial operation, we debrided the dead skin, tissue, muscle, and bone from the jaw. Metal arch bars with tiny hooks, regularly spaced, were placed around the upper and lower teeth. Later, small rubber bands would be attached vertically to hold the jaw in proper alignment during healing. The patient would be nourished either through IVs or a straw. Then we created what is termed a delayed skin flap by making two vertical parallel incisions eight inches long and four and a half inches apart on Walt's upper chest, and undermined the tissue beneath it. If we left it in that state until the next operation, the arteries and capillaries in the flap would enlarge, increasing its chances for survival.

It was two weeks before the next stage in the repairs. Again, with the patient under general anesthesia, we placed heavy metal pins through the two segments of the jawbone to stabilize it and bridge the gap, and attached the arch bars together. Then we cut around one end of the skin flap, lifted it off the chest, and stitched its upper portion over the chin wound. The unused portion of the peninsula of skin spanning the distance between the chest and chin was temporarily closed like a tube, protecting the raw side to prevent oozing and infection. Using a split thickness of skin from the boy's thigh, we covered the bed of the donor site on the chest. Then, as a final procedure, the shoulder wound was grafted.

For three weeks Walt had to live with his head tilted slightly downward, his chin connected to his chest via the flap. After that, we judged that the transferred tissue would live and had adhered sufficiently — and it was back to the operating suite, where we severed the flap and replaced the unused portion.

We had done the best we could. All in all, Walt was lucky. While the gunshot had fractured the jawbone, not enough was shot away to disrupt its continuity. Luckily, no significant nerves are present in that region, so his facial expression and speech were unaffected. Possible infection and other life-threatening aspects had been overcome. Actually, the only disfigurements were permanent cosmetic defects. The three-inch patch on his chin would always protrude somewhat and have a different color from the area surrounding it. People airily refer to "skin tone" as if it were all one color, but all portions of the anatomy vary greatly in texture and hue. And when Walt's beard began growing, the difference would be even more noticeable, for hair-bearing and non-hair-bearing areas could not be matched. He would always have the two unsightly scars on his chest.

It is estimated that there are nearly fifty million guns in this country and two and a half million new ones are purchased each year. Two hundred thousand people annually are maimed by guns. Half of these victims are nineteen years old or younger. I wish all opponents of gun control could be forced to sit in the Emergency Room of a major hospital for just one week. But Americans believe in their right to own and play with their lethal toys.

Well, let them play on. All I can do is try not to be sick as I put the pieces back together.

Chapter Ten

ALTHOUGH THE CLINIC was open on December 24, the case load was light because of the holiday. Celeste Bigliani, my very first patient, chose this morning for her final visit to make sure all was well. And it certainly was. The rhinoplasty had given her a normal-sized nose, which now gave her a perky look. Even her personality had changed; she was bubbly and confident.

"Satisfied?" I asked, after completing the examination.

"You bet!"

"What does your family think?"

"I guess they're reconciled to it." She gazed at me for a moment. "Can I ask you something?"

"Sure."

"Would it be possible — you know — after a nose like mine is done — to, uh, well — to change it back to the way it was?" The look on my face was so stunned, so disbelieving, that she hurried on. "Oh, no! It's not what you think! Not me! No way!!" She paused, gathering her thoughts. "I know it's been a long time, but when I first came in, do you remember Mama mentioning my brother Berto?" I nodded slowly, recalling the incident. Mrs. Bigliani had used Celeste's brother as a glowing example of a family member who was proud of his large hooked Roman nose — who looked upon it as an ethnic badge of honor. Celeste then began telling me a story that boggled the mind.

The Bigliani family was a wealthy one, its riches garnered from a lucrative olive oil importing business. Patriarch of the fortune was Celeste's and Roberto's grandfather, who ran the business with an iron hand from his residence in upstate New York. Berto was in charge of the family's sales operations in the southern states, and while he managed to get home infrequently, when he finally did, the first thing he saw was Celeste's redone nose and her spectacular new and attractive appearance. He was impressed. Without telling a soul, he sought out the best plastic surgeon in his area and had a rhinoplasty on his own. The overall result was great. The future looked bright. His appearance was vastly improved. The business was doing well and, along with everything else, he knew he was heir to his grandfather's six-million-dollar fortune. He always had been.

Then he was summoned to New York for a family reunion. And I guess all hell broke loose! Grandfather Bigliani, of the old school, took the nose job as a personal affront to him and to all the Biglianis who had gone before. One thing led to another, and the old man retaliated by calling his attorneys and disinheriting Berto. In desperation, Celeste said, Berto had been making the rounds of plastic surgeons, trying to find one willing to put the hump back on and restore his nose to the original state.

"He told me to ask you," Celeste concluded, "would you do it? I'm pretty sure he just wants it until Grandpa dies. Then he'll have it changed back again."

I looked at her, fighting the urge to chuckle. But six million dollars is no laughing matter. Still ...

I shook my head. "It could be done, I guess, with a silicone implant. But ethically — well, I just couldn't do it. You see, it falls under the category of an 'unreasonable request.' "

"An unreasonable request?" she repeated in puzzlement.

I nodded. "Let me give you an example. A couple of weeks ago a young black girl came to the clinic. She was really into the heritage thing. You know what I mean — her hair was done in corn rows, and she was majoring in Black Studies. She'd read *Roots* and had spent months tracing her tribal lineage. For reasons of her own, she wanted an ornamental bone put through her nose — she *had* to have it — and she wanted my help. I respected the deep pride she had in her race, but the way I see it, no matter what, a bone through the nose is an unreasonable request. I turned her down. Do you understand?" Thoughtful, Celeste nodded. "I'm sure your brother can find someone to do what he wants," I added. "It's just — well — not me."

Since it was Christmas Eve, I finished work at noon and frantically started my Christmas shopping. The stores, which looked as if they'd barely survived a hurricane, would close at six, so I had only hours left to make my selections from depleted stocks, aided by very tired and harassed sales clerks. I cursed my procrastination, but I did it every year, somehow convincing myself that if I waited long enough, everybody else in the world would have finished their shopping and it would be a breeze. It never worked out that way. I didn't even have a legitimate excuse. I'd had plenty of time; the month of December had been slow. Most plastic surgery is elective, and very few people choose to have operations just before the holidays.

Patsy's three sisters had flown out from Michigan to spend a few days with us, so I wanted to get gifts for them as well as my wife, and little remembrances for certain members of the hospital's staff, which I would pass out tomorrow with a special Merry Christmas. It was five minutes after closing time when I'd paid for and picked up the last gift-wrapped package.

Heading for the parking lot adjoining the store, I paused for a moment to admire the giant lighted Christmas tree perched high on the roof and to take a last look at the beautifully decorated and animated display windows that ringed the ground floor of the shopping mall. Turning, I practically ran into one of the many uniformed guards patrolling the parking area. Besides his regular service pistol, he was carrying a shotgun. It struck me as so incongruous that I guess the shock and surprise I felt were mirrored in my face, because he shrugged. He raised his voice so I could hear him over the Christmas carols blaring from the loudspeakers mounted outside the building.

"Had two attempted rapes, a mugging, and couple of purse snatchings last night," he said almost apologetically before he moved away.

Depression settled over me, for, like the story of Scrooge, it was a harbinger of things to come. Only a portion of the citizens of the city would be embracing the "Joy to the World" and "Peace to All Mankind" spirit the Yuletide represented. Another contingent would be maniacally determined to make merry in bars and at office parties. Drinking would erupt into vicious brawls and serious auto accidents. Tension would incite violent family quarrels. Strings of Christmas lights would short out, causing fires. The lonely and the depressed would attempt suicide; some wouldn't succeed.

And between now and New Year's, I would get my share of the victims to repair as best I could.

As I suspected I divided my time for the next week between various holiday parties and answering Emergency Room calls.

The first case was a lulu. Gus Rodman, who worked for a construction firm in a nearby valley, had been in a hurry to get home and share with his wife the good news of a hefty Christmas bonus. The city has several

186

winding, two-lane, mountainous roads that connect the valley with the city proper. Gus had decided on the one that might have the least traffic. With his head filled with visions of sugarplums, somehow he had inched over the double line on a blind curve, and was unfortunate enough to meet head-on another driver who had also allowed his attention and his car to drift on the steep turn. Moments later, that section of the road looked like a junkyard specializing in Toyota and Volkswagen spare parts.

Mr. Rodman was rushed to University Hospital's Emergency Room, where Dr. Frank Austin, a member of the Oral Surgery staff, did the initial examination. He determined that the victim had a compound fragmented fracture of the left elbow, a tongue that was almost cut in half, and a broken jaw. A major laceration just below the nostrils had lifted all of the skin and soft tissue of the nose completely away from the tip cartilage and underlying bones — bones that were unbelievably fragmented. Mr. Rodman's upper lip was cut and embedded with many slivers of glass. Pieces of flesh were hanging loose, and the lining inside his mouth was gashed so badly that one could look directly into his nasal cavities.

Dr. Austin scheduled the patient for immediate surgery and asked the E.R. staff to place hurry-up calls for an orthopedic surgeon, a plastic surgeon, and a dental intern to help. A combined effort was in order, and all three of us dashed into the locker room within five minutes of each other.

In the Operating Room, it took Dr. Austin and the dental intern over an hour just to get Mr. Rodman's tongue back together, while Alberto Mendez, from Orthopedics, tackled the repair job on the arm. Piecing the nose and lips back together was an extremely complicated procedure, and I began the time-consuming task of removing debris, glass, dirt, and dead tissue from the wounds. Then I started taking the pieces of skin, one by one, and placing them in proper alignment. Getting the nose and lip back in place was no mean feat, and it must have taken over a hundred and fifty stitches to do it. Dr. Mendez had just finished his procedure on the elbow, and I was just starting to squeeze the broken nasal bones into position, when Dr. Austin came back into the room.

"How much longer on your end?" he asked. I glanced at the wall clock. We had been toiling for almost three hours.

"Another hour, anyway," I said.

Frank nodded. "He's been under a long time. What would you think about postponing the jaw repair for a couple of days?" he suggested. I glanced at the anesthesiologist, who indicated his concurrence.

"Probably a good idea."

Before Dr. Austin left, he thanked me profusely for coming in on such short notice. Exactly how grateful he really was would be demonstrated a little later when he claimed Gus Rodman for his Oral Surgery Department and repaired the jaw himself. Like death, I guess, jousting for patients never takes a holiday.

It was after midnight — already Christmas Day —

and I was tired, but I decided to look in on the Emergency Room before leaving. Maybe I could circumvent the possibility of barely getting home before I was called back. I made my way through the swinging doors into the E.R. waiting room, which was crammed with dozens of patients, flanked by friends and families, clamoring for treatment. Pushing my way through to the examining area, I was met by pandemonium. Every cubicle was filled with the ill and injured. Doctors, nurses, interns, orderlies, ambulance attendants, and police officers were darting here and there as if they were in a Mack Sennett comedy. It was the busiest night of the year. Doctor William Devaney, the E.R. doctor, caught sight of me and hurried up like a thirsty man spying an oasis.

"Jesus," he snapped, "it's been like this since five o'clock. Can you give us a hand with the patient in bed three?" Without waiting for a reply, he sprinted off.

Even before I entered the examining room, I could hear the sound of a contralto singing "Jingle Bells" at the top of her lungs. Lying on the table was a buxom, motherly-looking woman. Blood was streaming down her face, but her arms waved like a symphony conductor's, keeping time with the carol. I leaned over, attempting to judge the extent of her injuries, and she suddenly enveloped me in a giant, paralyzing bearhug, pulling me down on top of her, bussing me with the wettest, slobberiest, bloodiest kiss in all history.

"Doc," she crooned, "I love ya! Merry Christmas!"

By the time I got untangled, I was smeared with blood and resembled a casualty myself. I glanced up to see Margie, one of the E.R. nurses, standing just inside the curtains, weak with laughter. Recovering, she helped me clean up the patient and I was able to see the multiple cuts on her face. Most were shallow and superficial; two or three needed stitches. While I sutured, I was able to get Mrs. Sperry's story. She'd been drinking with her boyfriend in a neighborhood tavern. When they were ready to leave, her escort had gallantly offered to get the car and bring it around. As she waited outside the bar, someone inside had heaved a beer bottle through the window, and the flying glass had showered over her.

Mrs. Sperry took up her song again as soon as I'd finished. It hadn't taken long, but by the time I stepped out of the room, the hectic pace of the E.R. had doubled. Patients were being shuttled in and out, but every time one was either admitted or released, there seemed to be five more waiting to take up the space just vacated.

To an outsider, it might have seemed chaotic, and I suppose it was — but there was an underlying orderliness and a contained efficiency among the medical staff. Most of them were old-timers, unflappable — they'd been through it before.

All except Dr. Ronald Cosgrove. A tall, lanky intern, Ronnie had been assigned to the Emergency Room just a few days before. Although he was ever so eager to please, his bewildered attitude made it clear that the holiday frenzy was something he had not been warned about in medical school. Instructions and requests were being snapped at him from every side.

"Dr. Cosgrove!" The authoritative voice of Dr. Devaney came from examining room five. "I need you in here — stat!" As the intern took a step in that direction, he was blocked by a nurse, who thrust several vials of blood into his hands.

"Take these to the lab — and hurry!"

An ambulance attendant stuck his head through the sliding door. "Doc — Dr. Cosgrove! Can you give us a hand out here?"

"Where's that orderly with the wheelchair, dammit! See if you can find him, Dr. Cosgrove!"

"What happened to the gunshot wound, doctor? Where did he go?" a police officer asked accusingly.

Ronnie's eyes were becoming wild and glazed as he struggled to accommodate everyone at the same time.

Ronnie Cosgrove was several years younger than the other interns. A precocious kid with an IQ bordering on genius, he'd finished high school at sixteen, gone on to his medical studies, and was graduated near the top of his class. Academically, he was sharp, but when it came to personal relations or sensitivity, he had a lot to learn. Every medical center has a walking faux pas, a perennial foot-in-the-mouther. At University Hospital, Ronnie was it.

For instance, while he was on that service, he attended a lecture by the Chief of Psychiatry, the subject of which was "The Psychodynamics of Adultery." In the middle of it, Ronnie stuck up his hand.

191

"Doctor," he asked, "are you speaking from personal experience?"

The audience roared but, unbelievable as it sounds, poor Ronnie wasn't trying to be funny.

Ronnie was not without wit, however. A bunch of us were sitting in the doctors' lounge one night, shooting the bull. Ronnie was complaining about how the interns always got the lousiest jobs to do in any department — that the "scut work" always seemed to fall to him. Then, somehow, the topic of discussion changed to sex. One resident idly wondered how much work it was and how much pleasure. He asked for opinions.

"I'd say it's fifty percent pleasure and fifty percent work," the chief resident said.

"Naw," Boyd Falmouth contradicted. "If you ask me, it's seventy percent pleasure and thirty percent work." Another doctor voiced the thought that the split was more like sixty-forty. There was silence for a moment, and then someone asked Ronnie for his opinion.

"It's a hundred percent pleasure and no work," he said with conviction.

"No work at all?" we asked in unison.

"Nope. Because if there was any work involved, you guys would have me doing it for you."

Anyway — that was Ronnie Cosgrove. Even as I watched, the bedlam in the Emergency Room increased. At least half a dozen persons were simultaneously shouting instructions and orders to the harassed intern as I walked out of the waiting room and paused to wish the E.R. receptionist a Merry Christmas.

I was just about to leave when the door between the examining area and the waiting room was flung open and Dr. Cosgrove catapulted through. He had obviously reached the breaking point. He glanced around wildly at the waiting horde of people, his hair mussed, his clothing blood-spattered, and threw up his arms.

"I don't know what the hell I'm doing!" he yelled — and then darted back inside.

A number of the startled, waiting patients who witnessed the performance suddenly began evacuating the Emergency Room. Either their complaints weren't as serious as they'd thought — or they'd decided it was safer to seek medical help elsewhere.

I made rounds Christmas morning. The Plastic Surgery Department had only a few in-house patients, and it didn't take long. I spent another hour distributing gifts to certain staff members of whom I was especially fond and amassing a pile of packages in return. I worked my way along, ending up at the Emergency Room.

Entering, I was aware of a buzz of excitement. Bryan Brooks, the handsome, swashbuckling hero of countless movie epics, was in a low-keyed argument with Dr. Devaney. Anita Brooks, the star's attractive, petite, auburn-haired wife, stood beside her husband, holding a folded, lace-trimmed linen handkerchief to an area just below her left ear. From snatches of conversation that reached me, I understood that Mrs. Brooks had stepped out on the patio, and a loose brick had caused her to lose her balance. When she'd fallen, the pointed corner of a metal chair had punctured the skin.

"I don't want you to sew it up, Doctor Devaney," the performer insisted. His tone was quiet, but held the underlying assurance of a man who *always* got his way. "Our family doctor's out of town, but I talked to him. He said to get a plastic surgeon. And I don't want just *any* plastic surgeon. I want the best! The Chief of the Department! Is that clear?"

Dr. Devaney nodded tightly, and with an almost imperceptible eye movement, indicated I should follow him into his office.

"It's barely a scratch, Don, and he's being unreasonable," he said, trying to mask his irritation. "I told him you were available and qualified, but I don't think he'll buy it. What he wants is Dr. Mayo or Jesus Christ."

I shrugged. "I'll talk to him if you want me to, but why don't you give Parmenter a call and see what he thinks?"

Devaney agreed, and a few minutes later he was explaining the situation to the Chief of Plastic Surgery. He listened a while before hanging up.

"Dr. Parmenter isn't too happy about it — but he's on his way. Brooks is news, and any time he's crossed, he uses it as an excuse for a press conference. That kind of publicity we don't need."

I stuck around, interested to see what would happen when arrogance met arrogance. About twenty minutes later, Parmenter appeared, deliberately parking his Jaguar in a prominent spot. I noticed that he was shaved and impeccably dressed in a suit that screamed wealth and prestige. Unintimidated, he strode up to Bryan Brooks, shook hands, and crisply introduced himself.

"I want the best for my wife," the superstar drawled. "Are you any good?"

Parmenter didn't even bat an eyelid. "Mister Brooks," he said evenly, "I'm not only the best plastic surgeon in this town, but I'm probably the best in the whole goddamned country. Maybe the world!!"

With that, he guided Mrs. Brooks into the treatment room. In less than five minutes he had sewn up the tiny laceration; it had taken only three stitches. Then he marched up to where the actor was busily signing autographs for the nurses.

"I'm finished, and your wife is fine. That will be five hundred dollars!"

I waited for the explosion, but Brooks promptly whipped out his wallet and extracted a number of large-denomination bills, which he handed to Parmenter. Then with a protective arm wrapped around Anita, he accompanied her to their waiting limousine.

Parmenter strolled over to the receptionist. "Deduct the standard amount for Emergency treatment," he said, "and donate the balance to the Needy Children's Fund."

He turned and grinned at me. "You find Santa in strange places," he chuckled. "Merry Christmas!"

When I returned home, everything was a beehive of activity. Patsy and her three sisters were in the kitchen, wrestling with the turkey and all the trimmings. When

I asked if I could help, there was a chorus of nos, and Patsy's voice was louder than the rest. It is a fact that a surgeon must protect his hands. Not just major injuries, but even a cut or a scratch could be troublesome. Any open wound is a potential breeding ground for bacteria that could be transmitted to surgical patients. Granted, I wore gloves when operating, but gloves have been known to break during a procedure. Any mishap, and there'd be no surgery for me for the duration. Patsy was more protective than I was. She had hammered in the nail that supported the Christmas wreath on the door, and had even sawed off the trunk of the Christmas tree herself so it would stand even.

When dinnertime came, she reluctantly agreed to let me carve the turkey and then left the room. She always did this. At first, I thought that the sight of the knife so close to my fingers unnerved her. That wasn't the case. She finally admitted that the way I approached the job made her squeamish. I'm afraid I carved in much the same manner as I operated — delicately cutting through the skin, carefully judging the anatomical joints, and slicing slowly with concentration and precision.

After everyone left, Patsy and I sat talking for a long time. This Christmas was especially meaningful for us. Even though we wanted a baby more than anything, we also realized that this would be the last Christmas we'd be alone — just the two of us together.

December thirty-first was one of those sunny, picture-postcard days for which our region is famous. But around four in the afternoon, fog began rolling in from the ocean and each hour saw the dense haze moving farther and farther inland. By nightfall, visibility was about fifty feet. I shuddered. With the mass exodus of celebrants wending their way from party to party on the clogged streets and freeways, there would be multiple accidents. And the fog would compound the problem.

The first casualty was Patrick Ebert. Astride a Harley-Davidson, the twenty-two-year-old youth had been heading for Pasadena to stake out an advantageous site from which to view the annual Rose Parade. The heavy mist had deposited a layer of moisture over the normal oil slick that coats the city's roads, and on a treacherous parkway, three cars had piled up in a minor fender-bending altercation. Because of the fog, Patrick had seen the obstruction too late. Three of his buddies, also on motorcycles, had been behind him, but they had swerved in time. The trio had trailed the ambulance to University Hospital.

I got the call.

All things considered, Patrick was comparatively lucky. Because of the road conditions, he'd been barely moving, and he was heavily padded with warm clothing in anticipation of the night's chill. He had a badly twisted bike, some bruises, a few superficial facial lacerations, and a broken jaw.

The one complicating factor was revealed as I examined the patient. The normal way to stabilize the jaw after setting a fracture is to wire the upper and lower teeth together until the bones have healed. But Patrick had no upper teeth, no artificial plate — just gums. It surprised me because he was so young, and I questioned him about it.

His eyes widened. "Good God, doc," he moaned. The Xylocaine I had injected had numbed his face, and he raised his hand to confirm the absence of his teeth. "A while back I had to have my upper teeth pulled. Pyorrhea or something. I just got my plate last week. What in the hell happened to it?"

"Let me check with your friends. They're waiting outside."

I explained the situation to the three concerned young men sitting in the reception area.

"He had his teeth in when we started out," one of the boys said. "I know he did! They must have popped out when he cracked up his wheels."

There was silence for a moment. "Look, doc," one of the others offered, "would it help if we went back and tried to find it?"

"You bet it would," I said. In the absence of teeth, hooks can be inserted in a patient's dental plate. Then by the use of suspension wires to secure the artificial plate to the maxillary bone, the jaw can be stabilized.

They hurried out, actually relieved that there was something they could do to help.

Within an hour, they had returned. Jack, who seemed to have taken charge, entered the E.R. triumphantly waving an intact upper plate like a banner.

"We found it!"

"Great." I handed it to the nurse, who would see that it was delivered to our prosthesis department for the necessary drilling of holes and inserting of hooks. "Did you have any trouble?" I asked.

They looked at me and everyone laughed.

"Well," said one, "let me fill you in on the scene, doc. When we got back there, we made a couple of swipes up and down the road, using our headlights. No teeth. We decided to park our bikes and go through the ivy along the side of the road, inch by inch. Right in the middle of all this, a police car glides up and the cops demand to know what in the hell we're doing. I guess they thought we were burying a body or maybe planting bombs along the freeway. So Jimmy here — he says: 'We're looking for some teeth, officer. How about some help?' "

Jimmy responded to the limelight with a smirk. "The fuzz ain't got no sense of humor."

"I thought they were going to run us in," Jack continued. "So I started to talk. I put on my sincere face and boy, did I talk! But just then, Eddie found the plate. They made all three of us open our mouths to make sure it wasn't ours."

Jack let out a loud, contagious guffaw. "Jesus, I'd give half my life to see a copy of their report on this one — 'Apprehended three suspects looking for teeth.' "

Coincidentally, the next patient brought in had similar injuries and, oddly enough, similar complications. Only the circumstances were different.

He was old and frail and he had been severely beaten. Those were the first things I noticed about Mr. Carl Woodrow. And his cheek and jaw had been broken. The elderly gentleman had already given the police a statement. He'd been on his way to a neighborhood party, only two blocks from where he lived, when he'd been mugged. A group of teenagers had piled out of a car, and attacked and robbed him. Their booty had amounted to a dollar and seventeen cents and a dime-store watch.

Surgically, Mr. Woodrow was a challenging problem because he had no teeth of his own nor artificial plates. He said that he'd been unable to afford dentures and had been too proud to seek public or welfare assistance. Besides, his meager pension made soft foods like cereals, bread, and milk the order of the day.

Society might be able to ignore Mr. Woodrow's economic and geriatric problems, but I was confronted with a medical one. The jaw fracture had to be set, and to do it, the bones had to be brought into proper alignment. So I admitted the patient and once again called on the hospital's prosthesis department. We agreed that they would take impressions and construct temporary dental plates — plates with no teeth embedded — and implant hooks so the necessary wiring could be done. It certainly was not as ideal a solution as using a person's own artificial dentures, which are carefully designed for proper fit and to compensate for bite — but they would serve the purpose. I also left orders for one of our social workers to look in on Mr. Woodrow and make available to him whatever help he was willing to accept.

I was crossing the examining area for what seemed to be my two thousandth trip when a distraught woman raced through the ambulance entrance.

"Somebody! Somebody, please!!" she pleaded. "You've got to help us! My husband! I think he's dying. Oh, dear God in Heaven, help me!!"

An orderly grabbed a portable stretcher, and he and a nurse dashed to the parking lot outside, with the woman leading the way. A few moments later they reappeared, flanking a tall burly Irishman — Dennis O'Brien — who was disdainfully denying any need for the gurney. His clothes were covered with blood and he held a crimson-soaked turkish towel to his face.

I hurried him into an examining room. He'd been stabbed in the abdomen, back, scalp, and left cheek. My primary concern was the abdominal wound, because that could be life-threatening, but there was no rigidity, no tenderness, and bowel sounds were normal. Indications were that the knife had not penetrated the peritoneum. Using a Kelly clamp, I probed and found that the cut was relatively shallow. All the wounds, in fact, were superficial except the one on the left cheek. It was C-shaped, extending almost three and a half inches, and went right down to the bone. Mentally I decided I had drawn another barroom brawl casualty. Judging from Mr. O'Brien's size and strength, I figured he'd been jumped by a small army.

"What happened?" I asked. "Who carved you up?"

"My wife," he said.

I was tired by now, and my tone was flat. "Any particular reason — or do you two have your own way of celebrating New Year's Eve?"

"I guess she had a reason. I stopped off to see my ex-wife before coming home. And my current ever-lovin' is the jealous type. She objected."

I remembered the frantic woman who had accompanied him. My patient was at least fourteen inches taller than his wife and outweighed her by a hundred pounds.

"So she stabbed you," I repeated. "What were *you* doing while this was going on?"

"It's a funny thing, doc. I just kind of stood there." He closed his eyes, reliving the incident. "I walked in and she was in the kitchen, hopping mad. 'I'm going to cut you, you bastard,' she says. Well, I'd had one or two belts, and I figured I'd call her bluff. So I unbuttoned my shirt, and stuck out my bare chest. 'Go ahead, you little bitch,' I said. And before I knew it, she was all over me with a paring knife. She said she'd fix it so my ex-wife would never want to lay eyes on me again."

Mrs. O'Brien had come close to carrying out her threat. The cheek laceration was dangerously deep and in the area of the facial nerve, which controls all the muscles — the movement of the mouth, the eyelids, the forehead — every expression. Tremendous deformity results if that nerve is severed. It is very difficult to repair, and decent return of facial function is unusual.

I held my breath as I tested him. He was able to

wrinkle his forehead, close his eyes, scrunch up his nose, and smile. Although no permanent harm had been done, it took me the next two hours to sew him up.

"Are you going to prefer charges?" I asked.

"Charges? Charges against Marcia?" he said incredulously. "Hell, no! She loves me! And I don't know what I'd do without her!"

As midnight neared, the pace became increasingly hectic. With the endless parade of patients, and with the entire hospital staff pushed up to and beyond the limits of capacity, I guess sooner or later a snafu was bound to occur. Even though I wasn't directly involved, it was newsworthy enough to mention.

A few minutes before midnight, a cab deposited Cecil Davis, a huge black man, perhaps twenty-eight years of age, at the E.R door. Well dressed and soft spoken, Mr. Davis explained that he had been in an argument in a bar and that someone had shot him. The bullet had grazed his right arm and then lodged in his abdomen. He was initially examined by the general surgery resident, who ordered abdominal X-rays, but because of the massive fat and muscular structure of the patient, the nature of the injury was difficult to determine. It was decided that an emergency operation was necessary to see how much internal damage had been done.

As soon as the incision was made, the bullet popped out of the fat just beneath the skin; there was no injury to the abdominal cavity itself. The recovery room was packed to the walls with patients, so Mr. Davis was placed in the Intensive Care Unit for observation, along with several other noncritical cases.

About four hours later, the members of the Detective Division of the Los Angeles Police Department descended on us in full force. Earlier that evening there had been a holdup attempt at the lounge bar of a nearby motel. Instead of complying, the manager had grabbed a gun from behind the bar and winged one of the pair of thieves. The wounded robber had shot back, killing the motel employee instantly.

Armed with descriptions from patrons, the detectives had traced the cab, and the driver remembered the rider. The destination had been University Hospital's Emergency Room. There was no doubt at all that Cecil Davis was their man.

Fascinated, I listened. By sheer coincidence, Patsy and I had occupied a room in that very motel only a few weeks before. For some time we had been seriously considering the purchase of a water bed for our apartment. It represented a considerable cash outlay, and we wanted to judge the advantages and disadvantages for ourselves. Bouncing for a few moments on display samples had left us undecided. Then, driving by the motel one evening, we saw that they advertised rooms with water beds, and we checked in for the night. We had a few drinks at the bar, and remembered the young manager with whom we had exchanged casual conversation. Now he was dead, his murderer was in my hospital, and probably right at this moment Patsy was lying on the water bed we had recently purchased.

The detectives demanded that the custody of Cecil Davis be turned over to them immediately, and began to arrange for his removal to the detention ward of County Hospital. They telephoned for an officer to guard him in the meantime, and then headed upstairs to read the patient his rights.

Whereupon all hell broke loose. Mr. Davis had simply disappeared.

During a reconstruction of the incident, one of the nurses admitted seeing a patient walking down the hallway near the Intensive Care Unit holding an intravenous bottle still attached to his arm. Hurrying on a possible lifesaving call, she had neither stopped nor questioned him.

The law enforcement officers were understandably furious. They didn't have to remind us that the state law required reporting the admission of anyone with a gunshot wound to the authorities. It was standard routine. In the hectic rush, I suppose everyone thought someone else had done so. How could a nurse not think it suspicious to see a patient from the Intensive Care Unit walking around holding an IV bottle? How had he gotten his clothes? In the I.C.U., patients are monitored constantly. How could he just amble out?

We didn't have the answers. We didn't even have any excuses. It was one of those bizarre situations that shouldn't have happened — that couldn't have happened — but did.

The story hit the front pages of every newspaper the

next morning. The reporters were scathing, and the hospital staff was severely criticized. We had it coming, I suppose.

I found myself scanning the front page and all the pages that followed. I read headlined articles and almost buried paragraphs. Nowhere was there any mention of the lives we had saved, the hours we had toiled, or even the backaches we'd sustained.

I guess there wasn't any place in the tabloids for our success stories. But during the short holiday span, a handful of dedicated people in University Hospital's Emergency Room had attended seventeen hundred and thirty-one human beings.

Chapter Eleven

A SHORT TIME after the holidays, this story almost came to an abrupt end. I nearly checked out of the world.

Three friends were going to Palos Verdes for some scuba diving. I was not officially on call and it was a beautiful Sunday, so Patsy and I decided to go with them. I had taken a scuba diving course and had been out four or five times on ocean dives. Recognizing my limitations, I had always stayed within a couple of hundred feet of shore and had never gone down more than forty feet.

Patsy, now eight months pregnant, settled herself on the sand with a book and my electronic beeper in her lap. I promised to surface regularly, and in case of an emergency call, she would signal me.

My friends were much more adept and experienced than I. I just followed along, and they kept going farther and farther out on the ocean floor, searching for the California clawless lobsters that are abundant in that area. I was having no trouble at all, even when we reached fifty feet, deeper than I'd ever ventured before. My equipment was working perfectly, and I had no difficulty adjusting to the new depth. I was having a great time, enjoying the errie sensation of being able to look up and not even see the surface.

And then I noticed that my air was running out. It wasn't too surprising, since inexperienced divers use up oxygen more rapidly. I switched to the reserve tank and signaled the others that I was heading back. We dive on a buddy system and are supposed to stay in close contact so that help is available if trouble arises. But I had five more minutes of air left, and I indicated to them that I was okay.

When I surfaced, I was shocked to find that we had gone out more than a quarter of a mile. I was equally dismayed to discover that swimming on the surface, weighed down with scuba gear, was extremely difficult. I hadn't gone more than a hundred and fifty feet before I realized that I was becoming unbelievably tired. I began to breathe rapidly. There were a number of things I could have done to ease the situation, such as merely diving three or four feet under the surface, where my equipment would have been no hindrance, but none of them occurred to me at the time. I struggled and slashed through the water, making agonizingly slow progress, working myself into a state of total exhaustion. I wasn't going to make it! It's a terrible feeling to suspect that you are going to drown.

I managed to raise myself in the water and waved frantically to Patsy, trying to convey my predicament. She gaily waved back, pointed to the beeper, and shook her head. There was no emergency.

The hell there wasn't! My arms were like lead weights. I had almost used up my reserve air supply, and it was becoming difficult to draw oxygen from the tank. I momentarily considered inflating my life pre-server vest, but while it would keep me afloat, it would also hinder my moving — and I was completely ob-sessed with feeling something solid under my feet. Finally, in a moment of desperation, I decided to drop my weight belt, which divers wear to descend into the water. Mine weighed twenty-two pounds. Even so, I hesitated. It was new and had cost twenty-five dollars. I shook my head. Idiocy! How in the hell could I equate a belt with my life? I unbuckled it and watched almost mesmerized as it glided off my waist and down into oblivion — an oblivion that could easily be my fate. That thought spurred me to greater efforts and I made a little progress, but the beach was still over two hun-dred feet away. Once again I shouted and gestured to Patsy. The roar of the surf drowned out my words, and she waved back.

Swimming the remaining relatively short distance was probably the hardest thing I've ever done in my life. Just as I was thoroughly convinced that I wouldn't make it, I looked through my face mask and saw the most beautiful sight in the world — the submerged rocks of the outer shoreline. Struggling with all my might, I finally made it to one of the boulders. I knelt on it, water still up to my neck, waves lapping over my face. After five minutes' rest, I managed to reach a slightly higher rock, and sat there half-dazed for a good fifteen minutes.

By moving from rock to rock, I made it. The experience had a profound effect on my professional life. My own determination and floundering terror came back to me later, each time I dealt with a patient facing the possibility of death. As they held on and fought with all their might, refusing to give up, willing themselves to hang on — to live — I understood.

Survival — it's wonderful.

It was survival that had motivated Joel Hampshire to lose two hundred and eighteen pounds. When I saw him at the outpatient clinic, he tipped the scales at a mere one hundred and eighty-five, down from his previous top weight of four hundred and three. From his history, it was apparent that he'd developed a severe glandular problem, which resulted in a tremendous weight gain. The glandular problem had been successfully treated, but his internist told Joel that unless he lost weight, his chances were bleak. Dieting didn't work, and it had been decided that the much publicized intestinal bypass operation was the solution.

Technically, this procedure is called ileal-jejunal bypass. The portion of the upper small intestine, the jejunum, is surgically attached to the lower part of the small intestine, the ileum. The end result is that the number of feet of the small bowel through which food passes, and where nutrition is absorbed, is greatly lessened. Thus weight loss inevitably occurs. Serious side effects from this procedure have been reported, and it should not be embarked upon lightly.

Joel had had the surgery about a year and a half prior to being referred to us, and he was proud of his new-found health and comparative slimness. But his skin had been tremendously stretched, and would never contract to hug his new body form. Large folds hung literally like pendulums on his abdomen, chest, arms, and legs, giving the appearance of an ill-fitting and baggy suit, ten sizes too large. He would need a number of operations to correct all of these areas, but he was most concerned about his belly. There were multiple rolls of excess skin dangling down from his lower abdomen. One was so extensive that it hung over and completely covered his genitalia. We scheduled him for an abdominoplasty, or belly-lift.

This is an operation that is relatively new, developed by a prominent South American plastic surgeon perhaps ten years ago. It was popularized as the "bikini operation" — so named because the scar is placed extremely low on the abdomen.

Usually they are done on women. The typical patient is fairly slender and is generally in better than average physical condition. She has one problem: pregnancies have devastated her lower abdomen. She has wrinkles and stretch marks, and the looseness of the skin gives her the appearance of having a paunch — all this in spite of the fact that she is not overwieght, watches her diet, and exercises religiously. While muscles can be tightened and toned, exercise will not help overstretched skin.

Since the procedure was developed, there have been a rash of articles in women's magazines extolling the benefits of abdominoplasties. The results are usually very pleasing.

But whether it is done on a woman or on a man — whether the problem is moderate or massive, the abdominoplasty technique is basically the same.

With Mr. Hampshire under a general anesthetic, we made a transverse incision across the entire lower abdomen, just above the pubic area, and began undermining the skin and fat from the muscles of the belly wall, working from the incision right up to the lower rib cage.

Although an abdominoplasty requires significant dissection, there usually isn't much bleeding, for there are only a few large blood vessels involved.

"Flex the table, please," I instructed my surgical nurse.

At this point, the patient's knees and shoulders are raised so that when the excess skin is removed, the edges can be stitched together without undue tension. I grasped the large flap of abdominal skin that had been created, pulled it downward over the incision, and marked the excess.

We were almost finished. A sterile gauze dressing was placed over the wound. Then we devised a so-called plate from the plaster splint material and laid it over the abdomen. Once that had dried, a five pound sandbag was placed across it. This would create weight on the skin and fat to make sure that they healed to the underlying muscles.

When I saw Mr. Hampshire that night, he was beaming but anxious.

"You're beautiful," I said, "but you'll have to wait a while to see for yourself."

I explained that he would have to stay in bed for forty-eight hours with his hips flexed. After that, I cautioned him to walk in a bent-over position for a few more days in order not to put unnecessary strain on the incision. Less than a week after the surgery, Mr. Hampshire was ready to be discharged.

I happened to enter his room as he was dressing to go home. He still had a tendency to stoop slightly, subconsciously protecting his surgical wound. He surveyed his new, smooth flatness with tremendous pride — and then slowly straightened. I saw him grimace for just a moment at the unsightly skin swinging from his arms, but when he left the hospital, he was walking tall, imbued with self-confidence and a new physical awareness.

"I'll be seeing you, doc," he called back.

I didn't doubt it for a minute.

Mrs. Baynes was back in the hospital. Almost a week before, she'd come to the clinic for her final check after the breast restoration surgery. There'd been no complications and everything was fine. As I had warned her, though, the breasts did not look absolutely normal. They were mounds with neither nipples nor the darker areas of skin — the areolas — that normally surround the nipples. But the difference couldn't be perceived when she was clothed, and her new contour was a vast improvement over her flat chest following the mastectomies. Early on, I'd explained the options of areola and nipple reconstruction, which are done as separate surgical procedures. During the examination, she'd asked me to run through the details once again and had made the decision then and there to go ahead. I had scheduled her for admission, and the first operation was booked for this morning.

Areola reconstruction is a skin-graft technique. The most commonly used donor site is the small inner lips of the vulva, since there is a similarity in color and texture. It's quite a simple procedure. We marked the exact spot on each breast where the areola should be located — a circle about four and a half centimeters in diameter. This was done while Mrs. Baynes was sitting upright rather than lying down; otherwise the positioning could be wrong. Under anesthesia, the small lips of the vulva at the entrance of the vagina were cut away and unfolded, and the incision closed. The catgut sutures would dissolve by themselves in ten days or so. Then we turned our attention to the circle of breast skin we'd marked. Freehand, with a scalpel, I completely excised and removed the outer layer of skin. No dermatome is precise enough for this and there is no margin for error. The graft was trimmed to fit the area and laid over it.

During sewing, the stitch ends are left very long. A sizable cotton wad soaked in mineral oil is put over the graft and the stitch ends are folded up over the cotton and tied across the top. This immobilizes the graft and helps it "take." We repeated the procedure on Mrs. Baynes's other breast and were finished. The dressings would be left on about four days, then I'd check to make sure the grafts would live — whether they had turned pink, indicating that a blood supply had developed. The recipient site is a good one, and we had never lost an areola graft yet. I was sure Mrs. Baynes would not be the exception.

Any doctor will tell you that sometimes a rash of similar cases will pop up during a relatively short period of time. For instance, a general surgeon may not get a gallbladder case for a couple of months, then suddenly he'll do three or four in a row. For me, late February was a time for repairing congenital anomalies.

Little Roger Nowacki was scheduled for surgery at eight A.M.

About two weeks before, Mrs. John Nowacki had brought her sixteen-month-old son to the Outpatient Clinic. The child's problem was a cleft palate, which results when in fetal life, the two palatine bones that grow in from either side and form the roof of the mouth don't fuse.

Unless it is corrected, there can be numerous problems. Feeding the child is usually difficult because of an inability to develop suction. Bottle nipples must have larger holes so the milk will drip freely, and care must be used to raise the infant so that the fluid will be prevented from backing up into the nose. More air than usual is swallowed, producing gas pains. Once the child is able to talk, the words may be distorted by inadequate pressure or by the sound of air leaking into the nose. While the cleft can probably be closed anytime before the age of four or five, it is a sound medical opinion that repair should be undertaken when the baby is between twelve and eighteen months.

The incidence of cleft palates is one in every six hundred and sixty-five live births, placing this congenital anomaly second only to clubfeet. In some families it seems an inherited trait. What it boils down to is that while we don't know exactly what causes cleft palates, we do know how to repair them.

Like many parents of children with birth defects, Mrs. Nowacki had a deep guilt complex, feeling somehow that she was at fault.

"How could it have been prevented, Dr. Moynihan?" she began our conversation. "I was so careful during my pregnancy. If I only knew what I'd done wrong!"

"The exact cause of clefts isn't known," I said, "but you can be sure it's nothing you did. A cleft is an accident — an accident in development. Nobody's to blame."

I went on to explain that the operation to correct a cleft palate consists of lifting the muscle and mucosa lining off the bones on either side, stretching the lining to the midline, and then stitching the two halves to each other.

I also warned her that even after the operation, we couldn't be positive that her son's speech would be normal. We wouldn't know until he was between two and three years old, and talking fluently. A lot depended on how much scarring occurred and on the mobility of the palate. If, in a couple of years, the boy's speech was mildly hypernasal, a course in speech therapy might correct it. If that didn't work, then later surgery, called a pharangeal flap operation, would probably improve it.

I headed for the locker room to change and begin my ten-minute scrub. I would be doing the cleft palate operation with Dr. Parmenter, and although he had not yet appeared, the scrub basin area was teeming with doctors. Most surgeons jousted for an early starting time, not only to save their patients the agony of waiting half a day with the terrors of surgery as their bed companion — but also because the surgeons preferred to operate when they were fresh and relaxed. Eight A.M. was popular.

Dr. Ronnie Cosgrove, the faux-pas kid, wandered through the area and spotted me. The weeks since the Emergency Room incident had not added to his tact. He paused beside me.

"Hey, do you know why surgeons wear masks?" He didn't wait for a reply. "Because the fees they charge are highway robbery! And do you know why they are anxious to start operating so early in the day?" Even though I wasn't sure what the punch line was, I'd gotten to know Ronnie, and I shot him a warning look — which he missed completely. "So they can get to the bank before it closes." His voice had inadvertently carried throughout the room and several of the nearby doctors glanced in our direction. I winced, lowered my head and raked the brush over my hands and arms furiously, hoping to shut him up. He stared at me, like a puppy waiting for attention. "Don't you get it?" he demanded.

Thank God, Parmenter joined me, and Ronnie scurried off, but the Chief of Plastic Surgery had overheard part of his remarks. He began to scrub.

"Was that young Dr. Cosgrove?" he asked curiously.

Wordlessly, I nodded. Parmenter shook his head. "Did you hear about what happened yesterday?" he inquired with a chuckle. "All of the residents were making rounds with Dr. Crenshaw, going from room to room, discussing cases. When they came to 503, it was Dr. Cosgrove's turn to present the case. As I understand it, the patient there is an elderly man who'd been struck by a car and had suffered multiple injuries. Cosgrove had boned up on the facts and was able to reel off the history and physical findings like a pro. The patient is doing okay, I guess, but seems to be recovering quite slowly. At any rate, Crenshaw asked your young friend if he had any opinion why the old gentleman was having such a prolonged convalescence.

" 'Yes, sir, Dr. Crenshaw,' he said. 'Five P's and a T.' "

Parmenter erupted with a burst of laughter. "Crenshaw's a pompous ass, and I can just see his face."

" 'P . . . P . . . P . . . P . . . T?' he repeated. 'Five P's and a T? And what might that mean, Doctor Cosgrove?' he demanded.

" 'Piss-poor protoplasm poorly put together,' sir."

"Jesus!" I murmured.

"Can't you just see Crenshaw?" Parmenter marveled. "He was dumbfounded. The residents were speechless. At least for a couple of seconds. And then somebody laughed, and then everyone did. Except Crenshaw. He just announced that the rounds were ended. I don't think Cosgrove even knew what happened."

The cleft palate procedure on Roger Nowacki went quickly and without complications — and that was good, because we had a full day in front of us.

Our next patient was fourteen-year-old Paula Linden, who had congenital alopecia of the scalp. Alopecia means baldness. Congenital, of course, denotes "present at birth." Its cause continues to mystify the medical profession.

Paula had been born and reared in a small town outside of Gallup, New Mexico. She had developed into an extremely pretty girl — except for the irregularly shaped hairless area some three inches wide by four inches long on the top of her head. Never allowing her daughter's hair to be trimmed or cut, Paula's mother helped her devise an elaborate style of swirls and bouffant puffs to cover the disfiguring baldness, but it took over an hour to arrange the complicated coiffure. Paula had managed to keep her affliction secret, but some of the other girls began teasing her for always wearing her hair the same way. So for a while she had worn wigs, but the inevitable day came when one of her classmates yanked the wig from her head. Paula had fled in tears — and refused to return to school. A student counselor suggested that the girl and her family consult a local surgeon. He had operated, and shortly afterward the family moved to our area.

Sometimes past errors in judgment catch up with the present, and I'm afraid that's what happened in Paula's case. I did not know the New Mexican surgeon, but I'm sure that he'd done what, in his opinion, was the best procedure. He had made an incision along one side of the bald area, taken out a strip of the hairless skin, undermined a portion of the normal scalp and pulled it over, advancing the hair-bearing tissue about one inch. He had told the Linden family that a similar operation, approached from the opposite side of the bald area, might do the trick.

We were dubious — and expressed our misgivings to the family. But they'd insisted that we proceed with the surgery.

With Paula under general anesthesia, Dr. Parmenter made the main incision and created a flap. We tried to extend this over the full width of the hairless strip, which was twice as wide as the area previously covered — but with all our efforts, it just would not stretch enough. If it had missed by only a little, we might have tried a fileting technique — making long, shallow incisions, accordion fashion, to stretch the flap more. We advanced it as much as we could, but there was still a prominent bald strip, and we were disappointed with the result. Some improvement had been gained, but Paula still had a bald strip.

Originally, the best solution might have been the popular hair-plug transplants. Maybe the surgeon in New Mexico was not adept at that procedure, or perhaps he was convinced that the "advancing" technique would work. I don't know. Unfortunately, I did know that the scar tissue from the two surgical procedures now delayed the hair-plug transplants.

It isn't exactly the easiest thing in the world to impart disheartening news to a family that has suffered through a problem for years. Nor is it easy to face a young girl who is extremely self-conscious and tell her that she must continue to live with her disfigurement.

Dr. Parmenter and I disconsolately agreed that it had not been one of our triumphs. As hard as we try, we can't win them all.

Microtia is a congenital defect that occurs once in every twenty thousand births. Medically, it is defined as an abnormal smallness of an ear. Six-year-old Peter Hughes's problem was officially listed as microtia, but he had been born with no left ear at all.

Giving Peter an ear required a number of operations, done in step fashion. During previous surgeries, we had first implanted a silicone prosthesis just under the skin, making a slit at the hairline and working the prosthesis down into proper position to serve as the skeletal framework. It exactly duplicated the cartilage of a normal ear, complete with the rim and all the convolutions and gulleys. As time passed, the skin adhered to this configuration. Then, three months later, we made a semicircular incision around the top, back, and bottom of the ear, freeing it from the side of the head except for the portion in front where an ear is attached to the head. A skin graft taken from the buttocks was used to cover the raw backside of the ear and the area from which it was lifted. The real trick had been estimating the proper size, for we had to keep in mind that the other ear would grow a little as our patient got older. The prosthesis, of course, would not. It might be argued that it would be better to wait to accomplish the reconstruction until Peter had attained his mature growth, but a disfigurement to a child just beginning school is a curse. It makes him the target of stares and the butt of hurtful questions from his schoolmates.

Since Peter had already had these operations, the reconstruction was almost finished. The purpose of the current surgery was the formation of the ear lobe, and we accomplished this with little trouble by creating a small skin flap behind the ear area and rotating the tissue into the position of a normal lobe and stitching it in place.

Many adults, after an ear amputation, opt for a purely prosthetic device. Maxillofacial prosthodontists have been able to sculpt ears of nonliving substances, realistically designed with wrinkles and skin texture, which can be attached by special, waterproof adhesives. There are drawbacks. They are expensive, and usually such a prosthetic device will last only between one and two years before it must be replaced. I also recently read about a middle-aged man who had lost an ear in an accident. Wearing a prosthetic replacement, the gentleman had been on an elevator when an attractive young lady entered. He had politely whipped off his hat and the adhesive gave way. The man's ear flew off, rolling to a stop at the feet of the woman — who promptly fainted in the man's arms.

Toward the end of the week, I was scheduled to do another congenital case with our "number two man," and just as I was starting to scrub, Dr. Burke joined me. Over the months, all animosity between us had disappeared. We would never be intimate friends, but he now respected my ability when we worked together, and I tolerated the quirks in his personality. Nevertheless, I was aware of one aspect of Burke's disposition: if he had a sense of humor, I had yet to discern it.

"Did you hear about young Cosgrove and the five P's and a T incident?" he asked indignantly. I hid a grin and nodded. "These kids they're sending us today," he said, "are a disgrace. They seem to have no reverence — no reverence at all — for the profession they've chosen."

I didn't reply. I guess every intern and resident, sometime in his career, gets to a point — a point brought on by the tedium of many menial tasks, con-

SKIN DEEP: THE MAKING OF A PLASTIC SURGEON

stant exhaustion, and the pomposity of his senior associates — where he has to do something to assert his independence. As Burke and I scrubbed away with the brushes, I recalled an incident that had occurred about three years before.

Surgical conferences are held at every hospital. Designed to teach, they are generally boring affairs, ritualistically held once a week, with residents presenting cases, including slides or whatever other exhibits might be pertinent, while the staff surgeons pontificate on the subject at hand. Unusual cases are the exception, and the stuffy atmosphere and droning voices are numbing.

My neighbors, the Rotowskis, had an English bulldog named Mister Magoo, who probably had the ugliest face that the canine world had ever produced. I was going through a phase of being a camera bug at the time and, fascinated, I had taken some 35mm slides of the pooch.

During one surgical conference, I decided to throw in a little humor. Maybe it was because I had been up thirty-six hours straight; maybe "the devil made me do it." At any rate, when it was my turn to present, I got up and said:

"My first case for presentation today is a sad one. The subject is a two-year-old male with multiple congenital facial abnormalities. He has drooping eyelids, a flattened nose, sagging jowls, a widened face, teeth that overlap, and floppy ears." For the first time in weeks, I noticed several surgeons straighten up in their chairs and begin to listen with full attention. "His family history is that he is an orphan," I continued, "born of

English parents, but adopted by a Polish family. I'd like your opinion as to what we may be able to do for him."

With that I flashed a color slide up on the screen. The doctors stared, and the delightfully ugly face of Mister Magoo stared back. Most of the physicians laughed, but several, like Burke, felt that my actions had desecrated the field of medicine.

We had finished scrubbing and as we made our way through the locker room, Burke stopped to chat with Dr. Crenshaw. While they were talking, the anesthesiologist passed by with a jaunty wave and entered the surgical suite. Crenshaw scowled in his direction.

It surprised me. Although movies and television depict the surgeon as the hero of the operating room, almost everyone in the profession recognizes the important part anesthesiologists play. Administering to the patient during the actual procedure is only part of it. Before the man with the blade ever appears, the anesthesiologist must check the gas in his machines, inspect the tubing, attach EKG leads, start an IV line, find an anesthesia face mask that is the proper size, tape a stethoscope over the patient's chest, make sure the patient is well oxygenated before administering the sodium pentothal, pass an endotracheal tube down the throat, and so on. His responsibilities are tremendous. Dr. Crenshaw's apparent antagonism baffled me.

"What time are you scheduled?" I heard Burke ask the other surgeon.

Crenshaw sighed. "Four o'clock. I hate starting this

late. And by the time you figure the A.F.A. time, it'll probably be more like four-twenty, dammit."

Burke chewed on that for a minute, unwilling to admit his ignorance. Was there a chemical equation with which he was unfamiliar? Had there been a new process devised? Finally, he couldn't stand it.

"What's A.F.A. time?" he asked. Neither man cracked a smile at Crenshaw's succinct reply.

"Anesthesia farting-around time! What else?"

Chapter Twelve

I N MID-MARCH, I had a rare privilege. I witnessed the
birth of my child.

When Patsy had first learned that she was pregnant,
several of our friends had touted natural childbirth,
extolling its many virtues and advantages. It sounded
good, and we had attended classes for the past couple
of months. We had gone to eight straight weeks of
lectures, read every pamphlet handed out, and had
seats in the front row for the several movies offered by
the group. Patsy had been especially diligent in practicing all the exercises and muscle-relaxing move-
ments. With me acting as the coach, she'd huffed,
puffed, stretched, squatted, and crouched with a vengeance. Hardly a day passed that we didn't exchange
encouraging phrases on how wonderful natural childbirth was going to be.

Patsy had been told by her doctor to expect delivery
around April second. It had been a long time since I

had personally delivered a baby — not since my intern rotation on obstetrics — and I decided to take a refresher course by watching a number of babies being born in the University Hospital's obstetrics wing.

One evening, about two weeks before our baby was due, I had scrubbed in on a delivery and was watching the obstetrician sew up the episiotomy when the charge nurse stuck her head in the door and told me there was a phone call from my wife.

"Don," Patsy said when I answered, "I don't feel well. I have a hunch those shrimp we had for dinner last night were bad. I think I've got food poisoning."

My wife was absolutely convinced that our baby would arrive precisely on April 2. Her obstetrician had told her — and that's the way it would be! She hadn't even considered the possibility of going into labor early. And to tell the truth, I hadn't given the possibility much thought either — until now.

"Are you throwing up?"

"No, but I've got these awful cramps. . . ."

"How often?" I asked.

"Oh, I don't know," Patsy said. "Let me see, I had one just when *Kojak* came on, and then — maybe about every three or four minutes."

I gulped. "I'll be right home. I have a feeling that little pack of food poisoning you're complaining about is going to want to get out pretty soon."

I raced to the apartment and checked her. Sure enough, the "cramps" were full-blown uterine contractions. Forty-five minutes after we arrived at the hospital, she delivered.

Natural childbirth. Maybe it works for some people — I don't know. In Patsy's case, what she had learned was of no use at all. Maybe it was because her labor was so fast that she didn't have time to use fully what she'd been taught. Then, again, maybe the whole concept is a lot of baloney. I thought back. Never once in all the lectures by the experts, or in anything we'd read, had there ever been any mention of *pain*. The fact is, the contractions hurt. They hurt like a son-of-a-bitch!! When you try to push a watermelon through a key-hole, no matter what the pamphlets say, it's going to hurt.

Patsy later told me that the second most wonderful moment of her life had come when the anesthesiologist administered the spinal block and the racking pain stopped. From then on, the delivery was a joy. The *most* wonderful moment of her life came when she saw our child. She watched the birth, fully awake, but totally free from pain.

I was in the room with her. It's a strange sensation standing beside your wife and watching your child being pulled from the uterus. When the baby was about three-fourths into the world, our obstetrician nodded in satisfaction.

"It's a boy," he announced. "Hey, Don, come take a look at your son."

It was as if I had suddenly turned to stone. After the past weeks of dealing with cleft palates, abnormal syndromes, and all the other birth defects, I was afraid. I didn't want to be the first to look at my child to see whether or not it was normal. I wanted someone else to tell me it was. I guess the obstetrician sensed my fears.

"You've got a beautiful son, Mrs. Moynihan — ten fingers, ten toes, and everything else in the right place."

I thrilled to the baby's first cry and took a peek. It's wondrous to look at a fully formed human being — a human being who'd been produced by two people, but who was now totally separate, an individual.

So . . . we had ourselves a son. We named him Trevor.

There was a humorous sidelight to our becoming parents. Moynihan is not a terribly uncommon name, I suppose, but its incidence is certainly not as widespread as, let's say, Smith or Jones. Yet, as luck would have it, Patsy's obstetrician had another patient with the same surname — one Sally Moynihan. The two women eventually had met in the doctor's waiting room, and to make matters worse, Patsy had discovered that her counterpart was due to deliver in the same hospital, during the same week.

From this coincidence, my wife developed a somewhat irrational worry — a fear that the babies would be mixed up in the hospital nursery, and that she would be given the wrong infant. No amount of reminding her about arm bracelets, footprints, and all the other safety measures employed to prevent mistakes did any good. When our child was born, the thought flitted through my head that at least, with his unexpected early arrival, we could relax on that score. Imagine my surprise when, as Patsy was about to be wheeled from the delivery room, the nurse daubed at her forehead and commented:

"It's all over, *Sally*. How do you feel?"

Patsy didn't answer, but her eyes widened.

"I want to see my baby," she suddenly insisted. "I want to see him right now!"

I watched her rivet her eyes on his face. Concentrating, she stared a long time — long enough so that she'd know that tiny face anywhere!

Spring seems to be the time for cosmetic plastic surgery. To many people, I suppose the approach of summer heralds pool parties, sleeveless dresses, upcoming vacations, increased physical activities — and maybe, subconsciously, rebirth — like the greening grass.

Bonita Steele was one of those women who had celebrated the equinox by taking a good, long look at herself in a full-view mirror. I saw her for the first time in the clinic.

"Darn it, doctor," she snapped, "I'm beginning to look like a *pear!*"

I wouldn't have put it quite so brutally, but there was no denying that my forty-six-year-old patient had a figure problem. She was actually a few pounds underweight, and her muscle tone was excellent, but she had what we call "riding breeches" syndrome — drooping buttocks and bulging hips that resemble a pair of jodhpurs.

Many women have a tendency to accumulate fat in these areas regardless of food intake or energy expenditure, and it is extremely difficult to get rid of the condition by dieting or exercise.

"Well, I'm not going to go through the summer ashamed to be seen in sports clothes," she said. "I've always considered large rumps stuffed into shorts or slacks a particularly unpleasant sight — and that's not for me. I read in a magazine about an operation. Do you know the one I mean?"

"Yes."

It was a fairly new technique, but I had done similar lipodystrophy procedures over the past year with uniformly good results. With the patient standing, the offending lumpy area is marked and then, under general anesthesia, long, wide, wedge-shaped strips of skin and fat, extending from the buttock creases to the sides of the hips, are excised. The competent surgeon is careful to place the incision in the gluteal fold, where it is unobtrusive and can be covered by a bathing suit.

"The procedure itself is relatively simple," I advised Mrs. Steele. "The most difficult part is the recovery period. No sitting as long as the stitches are in — and that's about two weeks. You can either lie down or stand up — but absolutely no sitting."

She thought on that. "How — how do you go to the bathroom?" she blurted.

"With difficulty," I said.

"No sitting at all — not for two weeks?" she repeated.

"Right. And it's very important. Until the wound heals, any sitting would pull on the incisions."

I saw the doubt appear in her eyes. "Gee, I have a husband and a pretty active social life. Sometimes I babysit — whoops!" — she grimaced at the use of the word *sit* — "with my grandchildren. I don't know. . . ." She felt her hips and thighs ruefully. "I hate the way I look, but . . . Well, maybe I'd better think about it."

I nodded my agreement. The inconvenient convalescence was the price for a slimmer silhouette. Only she could decide how much she wanted it.

"I'll let you know," she said before leaving.

Mrs. Steele was one of the few patients I never saw again. Over eighty percent of the people who consult a plastic surgeon for cosmetic reasons eventually go through with it. Oddly enough, it's a higher ratio than in general surgery, where a recommended operation may be lifesaving. Maybe it proves the premise that many persons value their looks more than their lives.

I would have estimated the age of my next patient — Chi Kyun Muncie — at sixteen. She was actually twenty-four, a stunningly beautiful woman with a dreamlike figure. Her manners and modulated voice attested to her upper-class Korean background.

She had met her husband during his tour of duty in Korea. There had been a whirlwind courtship and they had married. She confessed that her family had been extremely strict with her. They, like most of the Korean upperclass, had forbidden their daughters to associate with American servicemen. Except in rare instances, even high-ranking officers were looked down upon by such families, whose legacy of culture dated back centuries. Her relatives had refused to attend her wedding, but after seemingly endless red tape, she'd been permitted to join Lieutenant Robert Muncie in the United States.

So much for her background. As yet, I had been unable to discern any possible problem or defect. When she told me the reason for her visit to the clinic, I found it quite sad.

"My eyes," Mrs. Muncie said softly, "I would like them to be more — more Caucasian."

The major difference between Oriental and Caucasian eyes is that the upper lids of the former lack a skin fold. I was familiar with an operation in which a strip of excess skin is excised, just as in a cosmetic blepharoplasty. Then a small piece of muscle is removed and the desired fold is established by suturing the skin margins.

"I would also like my nose fixed," Mrs. Muncie continued determinedly. "As you can see, it is too broad — and too flat."

"There is nothing wrong with your eyes or your nose," I said. "What you're complaining of are ethnic characteristics."

"My husband does not like them."

I had never met Robert Muncie, but I felt an instant dislike. Sitting across from me was one of the most beautiful Oriental women I'd ever seen, and I couldn't help venting my annoyance.

"Would you be going to a plastic surgeon in Seoul with the same request?"

She shrugged and took refuge behind inscrutability, ignoring my question.

"Can you do it?" she pressed.

I knew we could. Yet, for the first time in many months, I asked my patient to wait, and sought Dr. Parmenter's advice. As I outlined the situation, he listened. When I'd finished, he gazed at me, slightly surprised.

"Well — so schedule her for surgery. What's the problem?"

"Dammit," I muttered, "the hell with her husband! She had the same eyes and nose when he married her. They didn't bother him then."

Goodnaturedly, Dr. Parmenter listened to my objections. An understanding smile appeared.

"Dr. Moynihan," he kidded, "also known as Crusader Rabbit, battling the ills of the world. I think maybe I'd better take a look and have a talk with Mrs. Muncie."

After a short chat with the prospective patient, our Chief quickly explained that we could and would effect the desired changes. He suggested we schedule the rhinoplasty first. Specifically, we would insert a silicone implant over the bridge of her nose to build it up, at the same time narrowing and moving the nostrils inward. At a later date, we would do the "Oriental eyelids" procedure.

I simmered down. Mrs. Muncie's problem wasn't all that different from a prominently hooked nose, I told myself. If it was making her unhappy, she had a right to have it altered.

The date for the operation was settled upon and Mrs. Muncie smiled gratefully and left. With all my rationalizing, I still wasn't too happy with the outcome. Had I been writing the script, her husband would have materialized with the assurance that he loved her exactly the way she was. But I guess that's not the way the world turns.

I drew several disturbing cases during this particular period.

One of the most dismal was Patrick Whitehall, a twenty-two-year-old quadriplegic. At the age of fourteen, the young man had been hit by a truck while riding on his bike, and in addition to numerous other injuries, his spinal cord had been severed. As a result, Pat was unable to move his legs and had very limited motion of his arms. Despite everything, he was extremely cheerful, bright, and ambitious. He had gotten a job in an electronics factory whose policy stressed hiring the handicapped. Pat inspected parts by means of a supersonic scope, dictating his finding into a specially rigged recorder. Our patient was proud of his usefulness and of his ability to earn a living. However, sitting in a wheelchair hour after hour had caused chronic recurrent skin breakdowns on the buttock and sacral areas.

Over the past years at regular intervals, twelve separate operations had been performed to repair the open, oozing ulcers. Simple skin grafts could not provide the necessary thickness for padding, and most of the procedures had involved rotating local skin flaps.

When I examined him, although the wounds were closed, the covering was dangerously thin. It was just a matter of time before he'd be in serious trouble. For our patient to continue to function, additional fat and skin must be provided over the bony prominences that were breaking down. Unfortunately, almost every square inch of available tissue had already been used.

There is an operation known as a total thigh flap that is a last resort in problems like this.

A last resort — because it involves amputation of a leg.

An incision is made right down to the femur, the large bone of the thigh, and all tissue, fat, muscles, tendons, and arteries are lifted from it, preserving them in one huge flap. Then that flap is folded up and over the back of the lower torso, providing adequate padding for the ulcerated areas. Finally, the stripped leg bone is cut off at the hip.

It seems like a horrendous operation, but as I hesitantly explained the possibility to Pat, his reaction was extremely calm and realistic. I was surprised that it took him such a short time to agree.

His philosophy countered my natural reluctance to removing the leg of a twenty-two-year-old man. Mr. Whitehall realized that without the operation, he was facing a lifetime in bed, flat on his back. He would not be able to sit, much less continue with his job. And as he pointed out, his leg was paralyzed and totally useless. In his eyes, the operation was not a mutilating or disfiguring procedure, but a positive step forward.

The operation went well, and we were able to supply massive tissue to cover the buttocks and sacral area. It would last a long time, but probably not long enough. Eventually, Mr. Whitehall's other leg might have to be used in the same manner.

Before I scheduled the surgery, I made sure that the hospital had a water bed available. They are a godsend to the paralyzed, where the pressure from a regular bed against bone is too great for the skin to tolerate.

I happened into Mr. Whitehall's room a few days later when he had a visitor, and was introduced to Matthew Patridge, a young blind man, whose seeing-eye dog lay quietly at his feet. He was a fellow worker at the plant, an electronics assembler whose intelligence and nimble fingers more than made up for his lack of sight. In the course of our conversation, I mentioned to Mr. Whitehall that he should exert every effort to purchase a water bed for home use.

Later I found out that our young blind friend had passed along my remark to his associates at the factory, and a collection had been taken up. Every employee had contributed. Management had made up the difference, and when Mr. Whitehall was discharged from the hospital, the newest model water bed was waiting for him at his residence.

The world is filled with kindness — counterbalanced by cruelty.

A few evenings later, when four-year-old Hubert Washington's mother brought him into the Emergency Room, I took the call.

The ugly third-degree burns on the child's buttocks were not fresh — I judged they were at least twenty-four hours old. I knew that split-thickness skin grafts would be necessary, so after attending to the child's immediate medical needs, I had him admitted.

Then I returned to talk to Mrs. Washington so I could get the required facts for the patient's history.

"How did it happen?" I asked.

"My husband was fiddling around with the car — you know, like tuning the motor? Well, when he started revving the engine, he didn't know that Hubie was standing in back of the car, right in front of the exhaust pipe."

I automatically nodded and wrote it down, but I noticed that the woman was reluctant to meet my eyes.

"When did the accident occur?"

"A little while ago — an hour, maybe."

I knew she was lying. The rest of my questions were answered with monosyllabic evasiveness. Later, I went upstairs and tried to question the boy, but he seemed too terrified to talk.

I sought out Dr. Devaney, who was in charge of the Emergency Room.

"About the Washington kid," I said, "did you notice anything odd about the burns?" Devaney thought for a moment, and I didn't wait for him to answer. "There's a pattern — like vertical stripes. You have to look close, but there are regularly spaced areas that seem to be more deeply burned than others."

"So . . . ?"

"The mother said the injury was from an automobile exhaust pipe — and that it happened right before she brought him in."

"No way."

"You know," I said, "the ridges in the vent of a hot air furnace could have caused that pattern."

"Or a steam radiator," Devaney offered. "But the kid would have to have been held against it by force." We were both silent. "Do you think we have another child-abuse case on our hands?"

We both knew that a normal parent will rush an injured child for immediate aid; however, abusers will wait until they become truly frightened or delay seeking help until they have concocted a logical explanation.

"I think it's worth reporting," I said.

"Right on," Devaney agreed. "We've had three battered-child cases already this week. What in the hell ever happened to punishing a kid by making him sit in a corner?"

It's a sociological fact that an increase in child-abuse cases always accompanies a national recession. There is a direct relationship between deliberate child injuries and unemployment. Many parents are anxious and frustrated over economic worries and, as a result, they develop a low tolerance for a crying or a mischievous child.

Our findings were sent to one of the hospital's social workers, who passed them along to the youth authorities.

The State of California has provisions demanding detailed reports of possible child-abuse cases, but they are often difficult to prosecute. Evidence is hard to obtain. Abusive acts are usually inflicted within the privacy of the home, witnessed only by a spouse, who has a legal right to refuse to testify. But at least Hubert's case was now a matter of record. If there was another instance of suspicious injury within the Washington family, the legal gears would begin to grind.

Statistics on child abuse are often misleading because many cases are not reported, or the doctor in charge is unsure of his suspicions. Still, in all, each year over five hundred thousand children — a half million — are injured because of deliberate abuse or neglect. The mortality rate is sickening, with the majority of deaths caused by skull fractures, concussions, burns, and injuries to internal organs.

I later learned that the authorities, although as suspicious as we, felt the evidence in the Washington case was too equivocal to take action.

Poor little Hubert would have to take his chances.

Chapter Thirteen

THE MONTHS SEEMED to tumble over each other. The routine was pretty much the same, but every day was different. One Wednesday morning started out normally enough, but there was a series of events with a significant outcome.

During rounds, Dr. Parmenter and I looked in on Mimi Crowley. We had performed a blepharoplasty on her the day before to remove the unsightly bags around her eyes. There was a running gag between Dr. Parmenter and me — we had seen more of Mrs. Crowley than we had some of our relatives. She'd already had a face-lift, a chin implant, a breast augmentation, and a tummy-tuck.

"How are you?" Parmenter asked, taking her hand.

"Fine, just fine," our patient said; then, with a grin, "You know, I was just lying here, thinking. If I keep this up, you can use my body for spare parts." We all laughed. She was a great patient.

As we were about to leave, Dr. Parmenter glanced at the woman with a heavily bandaged face who was occupying the other bed in the double room.

"Morning, dear," he said. "What happened to you?"

"Car accident," she sighed ruefully, "about six months ago. My cheek hit the steering wheel. It was all caved in — my cheek, I mean. They tried to fix it then, but it still looked kind of sunken and . . ." She floundered for a moment, then went on. "Anyway, yesterday I had — what do you call it? — a dermis skin-graft operation? To build it up."

I could see every muscle in Dr. Parmenter's body tighten. "Who took care of you?"

"Dr. Bogart."

"Uh-huh. And how do you know Dr. Bogart?" Parmenter pressed.

The patient shrugged. "I went to the General Surgery Clinic. A Dr. Crenshaw saw me and referred me to Dr. Bogart."

Dr. Parmenter practically yanked me out the door to the comparative privacy of the corridor.

"A facial depression!" he ranted. "With a dermis skin graft — pure and simple! *Nobody* can say that wasn't a plastic surgery case! And Crenshaw assigned it to Bogart in E.N.T. I wasn't even consulted!"

He paced a few steps and turned back. "If it's the last thing I do," Parmenter vowed, "I'm going to keep those E.N.T. men from stealing our cases!"

I knew I was hearing one side of a long-standing argument. There are many types of operations, particularly on the head and neck, that are cosmetic or reconstructive in nature and that plastic surgeons consider their domain. But they are also done by ear, nose, and throat doctors and also, to some degree, by oral surgeons. It's a source of great conflict.

"I don't like the pirating any more than you, but we can't bird-dog every case," I said. "I've got an idea, though. Maybe you could push through a general policy change so that all head and neck tumors are operated on by the general or plastic surgery departments. Those guys in E.N.T. don't even have a residency program, and there isn't a heck of a lot of that type of surgery coming through. What filters in should be utilized for training."

I saw that I'd lit the fuse to an idea. To Parmenter, it was a way to get even. I also knew that he shared a concern that worried me. At the end of every resident's training, the Chief of his department is obligated to fill out a comprehensive form, which finds its way back to the American Medical Association. On it is listed the various procedures each resident had done during the training period — the types of cases, how many, whether he was assistant or primary surgeon, and so on. It is a safeguard against hospitals offering residencies and not giving young doctors adequate training. Unless the exposure is up to snuff, official sanction of the residency is withdrawn. I was okay except on one count — I had done practically no head and neck tumor surgery — and if Parmenter wanted his department to keep its A.M.A. approval for future plastic surgery residents, we both knew I'd better get some experience in that specialty.

"It's not a bad idea," Parmenter mused. "I'll give it a try at the next staff meeting."

However, for the first time since I knew him, Parmenter's charm and expertise in getting his way failed. Dr. Crenshaw, Chief of Surgery, was a formidable adversary and he opposed the recommendation vehemently. While he recognized the merits of the argument, he was not about to allow bureaucratic suggestions to hamper his personal decisions or the power he'd acquired.

Later, Parmenter admitted his defeat.

"We're stymied — temporarily," he said. "There's just not enough head and neck surgery to go around in a private facility. Anyway, Don, as far as your training goes, I'll come up with something."

A couple of days later he called me into his office. "I've been thinking. What you really need is some Veterans' Administration Hospital experience. Anyway, I checked with the local boys, and for once they're fully staffed, but . . ." He went on to explain that a VA Hospital in an adjoining state was desperately looking for a surgeon to fill in for three months. "From what I understand," Parmenter ended up, "they see a lot of head and neck tumors — and they need all the help they can get."

It was a big decision, involving a temporary move. Patsy and I discussed it far into the night. Finally it was agreed that I should go. The facility offered a tiny bachelor apartment right across the street — fine for one, but totally unsuitable for a couple with a baby. Closing one apartment, finding another, and a complete uprooting seemed impractical for just twelve weeks. I would go alone — and we would commute on my weekends off, with Patsy either coming to see me, or vice versa.

But before I started my new assignment, Patsy reminded me that we hadn't had a real vacation for over three years. Our son was now old enough to be deposited with his grandparents for two weeks, and Dr. Parmenter agreed to my taking a short leave.

We took our holiday in an unlikely spot: Northern Ireland. Being Irish, I wanted a firsthand impression of the turmoil there. It was a trip like no other we'd ever taken. We were searched by the British Army. We saw a Catholic youth shot by soldiers. We watched Saracen tanks roar up and down the main streets. We hit Belfast on Orangeman's Day and watched an emotional six-hour parade. From Belfast, Patsy and I decided to rent a car and look up some long-lost relatives in Eire. They were intensely interested in the fact that I was a plastic surgeon, but weren't sure exactly what I did. I explained that I treated burns and birth defects and skin cancers. They were impressed. I should have stopped while I was ahead, for when I told them I also did cosmetic surgery, the oldest male member of the family shrugged.

"Well, I tell you, Cousin Donald. The way I look at it — if a person can't get through life with the nose

God gave him, maybe he doesn't deserve to be here in the first place!"

We arrived back home on a Friday night. Patsy and I spent a couple of days lazing, unpacking, and enjoying the reunion with our son Trevor. How can you miss a baby so damned much? He had grown into a beautiful little boy, with a mass of curly blond hair — almost a twin to the tot whose likeness appeared on the Pampers diapers box. Chubby, good-natured, and animated, he was truly a joy in every way.

Sunday was bright and warm, and I got an early start. By nightfall I'd reached my destination, and there was even some order in my new apartment before I went to bed. The weather held and the next morning, when I was due to report at the Veterans' Administration Hospital, was an absolutely perfect day. Instead of a pewter, smog-dimmed sky, it was actually bright blue, billowing with puffy clouds, and, although the sun was warm, a brisk breeze cut the heat. On a morning like this, I told myself, nothing could be bad.

The Veterans' Hospital had been erected about ten years before, but constant enlarging had resulted in numerous, sprawling, multistoried buildings, each painted a somber battleship gray, haphazardly and inefficiently strewn over many acres. For some reason, instead of the bright sunlight penetrating the facility, its warmth seemed to be held at bay.

As I drove through the gate, I saw countless elderly men shuffling along or passively sitting on gray benches or in gray wheelchairs placed beneath white-washed eucalyptus trees. During the daylight hours, the hospital patients were permitted to sit, lounge, lean, or totter outdoors. Intermingled with the oldsters were kids from the Vietnam war and other, now middle-aged, victims of the "police action" in Korea.

I knew a little about the basic organization of a VA Hospital. Most of the personnel are under Civil Service. However, it is policy to form an affiliation with a large nearby teaching facility, from which supportive medical talent is drawn.

For instance, the Chief of the VA Hospital's E.N.T. Department was also a senior staff member of the state's University Hospital, where he spent at least eighty percent of his working hours. The other twenty percent was devoted to administrative guidance, consulting, and twice weekly teaching rounds at the VA Hospital. The workload was handled by the senior resident, who was actually in charge, and a junior resident, who assisted him. Private physicians and staff doctors affiliated with other hospitals were available for special consultations or difficult surgery — for which they received a fifty-dollar fee from the government. The responding doctors viewed their services as charitable contributions, and a means of enhancing their academic standing. Most served cheerfully but, understandably, without special dedication.

After waiting an interminable time alongside the desk of a harried receptionist who obviously wasn't expecting me, I was directed through a maze of tunnels and hallways to the utilitarian office of the senior resident of the E.N.T. Service, Dr. Theodore Bentley. When he arose to shake hands, I saw that he was very thin, perhaps an inch or so under six feet, with closely cropped light brown hair. He greeted me warmly and lost no time at making a stab toward officially indoctrinating me regarding the problems I would be facing. It was a valiant attempt, but doomed. There was a constant stream of people in and out, asking quick questions, seeking advice, and requesting signatures on the thick, multipart requisition forms, without which government bureaus would falter and die. His phones rang constantly, and every sentence directed to me, or my reply to him, was interrupted at least two or three times by their clamor.

It became obvious that he had a number of cases on which he needed consultation or medical help. He methodically went down his list of available doctors, making call after call. None was available at that precise moment. He was transferred, he was placed on hold, he argued with answering services, he left messages. Eventually his calls were returned. The tenor of most of the conversations was similar.

"Dr. Whittaker? Good morning — this is Ted Bentley at the VA." He went on to describe the particular problem and his specific need for assistance. "Oh, you can't make it until a week from Tuesday?" Excuses and apologies were forthcoming from the other end. "I understand. But in my opinion, Mr. Mallon's condition is critical. I'll see if maybe Dr. Cameron might have some free time before then — if not, I'll call you back."

When he was finally successful in eliciting a reluctant physician's promise to come within a reasonable time, Bentley was noticeably elated, jotted a note on the patient's file — and began anew the time-consuming series of calls on behalf of another of his charges.

Almost an hour passed with Dr. Bentley talking on the phone and me listening, before the door burst open and Dr. John Anderson, the junior resident, strode in. I noticed that he hadn't bothered to knock. Even so, Dr. Bentley breathed a sigh of relief.

"Dr. Moynihan, meet Dr. Anderson." We shook hands. Anderson was about twenty-nine, short, squat, prematurely balding, with a certain aura of sloppiness about him. The senior resident seemed not to notice his colleague's shortcomings.

"John will show you around and get you settled in," he said, and with a friendly nod of dismissal, turned his attention once again to the stridently demanding phone.

Dr. Anderson left me sitting — deliberately, I think — while he selected, at random, several documents lying on Dr. Bentley's desk and perused them. While Bentley talked on the phone, Anderson made pointed suggestions to his superior, verbal comments and asides bordering on being critical. I was getting a taste of his personality — rude, officious, and argumentative. But I would be working closely with him, and I was determined to have it be a pleasant association.

He led me to the elevators and pressed the call button. "We might as well start with the top floor," he announced. As we waited, he deliberately studied me from head to toe. "What are your qualifications?" he asked bluntly. I ran through them quickly, touching the salient points.

"Well, in terms of surgical experience," he admitted, "you've got a hell of a lot — more than Ted and me put together." I saw the resentment flicker in his eyes. "But don't kid yourself; here, you're low man on the totem pole."

While resenting his crudeness, I realized he was probably right. It was the old story of leaving your own domain and power structure, and invading someone else's.

Anderson leaned on the elevator button again. "Damn," he exploded. "They're probably on their coffee break." I glanced at my watch. I had arrived before eight. It was now after ten. "Well," he said, "we either wait — or tackle the stairs. So we wait." He perched on the corner of a nearby table and indicated that I could do the same.

I stared at the bank of three elevators. "They all take their coffee breaks at the same time?" I asked. "Couldn't they alternate?"

"Look, boy," he sneered, ignoring the fact that I was at least five years his senior, "the Civil Service *Manual* says ten to ten-fifteen — and that's the way it is!"

"But if there should be an emergency . . . ?" I floundered.

"When you have a minute — *if* you ever have a minute here — look up Emergency under 'E' in the *Manual*. It's probably covered."

Before the end of the week, I would realize that the Civil Service *Manual* and the importance of "seniority," which it so carefully spelled out, was the guiding force. Whether it was an elevator operator, a lab technician, a clerk, or a janitor, status and power were held by those who had been on the Civil Service rolls the longest. There was little recourse against surly, inefficient service. These were people with institutional mentalities. As workers, they made a decent salary, their jobs were protected, and hours and conditions of work were strictly outlined. At the end of their rainbow was a generous government pension — not for the quality of service rendered, but for the length of time served. It was difficult to dismiss them — or even to reprimand them. Complaints against individuals involved endless paperwork and appearances before grievance committees and federal inquiry boards. They had immunity — and they gloried in it.

But I was still an innocent as we waited, and I don't know how long it was before one of the elevator doors opened. The operator still held a plastic carton of coffee and had just popped the remaining quarter of a doughnut into his mouth.

"Hiya," he greeted us. We patiently waited inside the cab until he'd finished, drained the last drop from the cup and basketballed the container into a nearby litter can. Informality was certainly the watchword here; it would take some getting used to.

"This is Dr. Moynihan," Anderson said. "First day — and I'm showing him the ropes."

"Ummm," mumbled the operator. "Up or down?"

"Up," the resident advised; "we might as well start with the Zoo."

He watched me for a reaction, and I managed to hide my distaste. I sensed that my tolerance was being tested by this brash young man.

The Zoo, as Anderson had indelicately called it, was two wards, each with twenty-eight beds — fourteen in a row on either side — with the two halves separated by a nursing station. This area, which housed most of the head and neck tumor patients, was probably the most depressing sight I had ever seen.

The smell of hovering death was a physical thing. I ran my eyes over the group in general. In the first bed was a man whose head was swollen to the size of an inflated balloon because of tissue edema from an uncontrolled cancer. Next was an elderly patient with what appeared to be a parotid gland tumor the size of a small cantaloupe. A seventy-five-year-old gentleman was attempting to read, his spectacles askew to protect the large antral carcinoma that had perforated through the skin of his cheek, resulting in a huge, open, oozing ulcer. Many of the patients tried to smile at me — and failed — because of facial paralysis from nerve injuries. Most of them had tracheostomies; some had laryngectomies and, if able to speak at all, were capable only of guttural, slurring sounds. They were constantly hawking up large amounts of foul-smelling secretions from their lungs, expelling the stuff from their tracheostomy tubes.

To hide my dismay, I went from bed to bed, mumbling a few words of introduction and greeting, glancing at chart after chart. I discovered the average ward patient's age was in the late fifties or sixties, although most seemed years older. I also became aware that most of them had waited too long — their malignancies were inoperable. All they could be offered was radiation therapy, a delaying process. From the charts, I saw that many had received such treatment without results, or had recurrence of prior tumors which were unresponsive to therapy. With possibly one exception, every single patient I saw was merely waiting to die. As we reached the end of our tour of wards, Anderson glanced at me.

"We've got the *really* sick ones in private and semiprivate rooms," he said. "Come on, I'll show you the way."

So I was introduced to the circle of bed assignments. Those who were treatable were kept in the wards. When death became imminent, they were moved to individual rooms. When the occupant of a private or semiprivate room was deemed in critical condition, the arrival of the hospital's chaplain signified that his bed, in the dignity of the private room, would soon be occupied by a worsening case from the ward — thereby freeing space for a new admission. The patients were familiar with the formula and could judge their prognosis and probable time of death accordingly. It was like a kind of lethal musical chairs.

When we had finally worked our way back to the nursing station, I met Mrs. McGrory, the RN in charge of the service. She was middle-aged, attractive, with a no-nonsense attitude. She knew her business and was highly efficient.

"Dr. Bentley called and left a message for you, Dr. Moynihan," she said. "He's on a tight schedule, and usually skips lunch, but he suggested you might join him in the cafeteria for a quick cup of coffee around one." We both glanced at the wall clock. There were five minutes to spare. She turned to Anderson. "He said you, too, doctor, if you're free."

"I'm running way behind," Anderson said shortly, "so I'll pass. See you later," he called to me.

Mrs. McGrory began the involved directions for finding the commissary. Seeing my growing confusion in the face of her instructions to go downstairs, turn right, turn left, turn right again, then one flight down . . . she ended up sketching a small map. Without it, I suspect I would never have been seen or heard from again.

I scanned the austere cafeteria without sighting Bentley and decided to take my place in the long line at the food counter. Having seen the patients, I had little appetite and settled for a cup of coffee.

I spied Dr. Bentley as he entered, and waved to get his attention. He joined me, and wasted little time getting down to the business at hand.

255

"You've seen the patients?"

"Yes . . . but . . ."

"I know what you're going to say," he interrupted tiredly, "and before we get down to specifics, let me fill you in. You saw the men in Ward A?"

"Yes."

"They're all tumor cases — that's why they're on our service. But twenty-one of the twenty-eight are chronic alcoholics. Anderson calls them bums. They're not, really — it's just that for some reason, they didn't seek early medical attention. So, we do what we can."

I shook my head. "It's like something out of the Dark Ages. With all the scare publicity about tumors and cancer, all the free clinics, how in the hell can someone ignore . . ."

Ted took a sip of his coffee and grimaced at the taste. "Look, help was available. You can't indict the system. Some of the men you saw just figured they could drink their tumors away. A lot of the others *have* undergone major operations, and then had a recurrence." He paused. "Do you know what 'dumping' means?" He didn't wait for a reply. "When there's nothing more that can be done, when the family is screaming for advice and guidance, the private physician determines whether his patient is a veteran. If he is — hallelujah! He has him sent to the VA Hospital for us to take care of in his terminal state. We call it 'dumping' — but I guess when you really get down to it, there isn't much choice."

I was silent, thinking my own thoughts. In this day and age, anyone who is ill, regardless of his finances, has some place to go. No city or county hospital will turn a patient away. They may bill, and attempt to collect, but if there are no funds to pay, that's the end of it. But even with all I'd seen, Veterans' Administration Hospitals were probably better than most public facilities. They were equipped to handle anything from acute illnesses to nursing care. Financial strength of the patient was immaterial. He need only to have an honorable discharge from some branch of the armed forces. Generally, the medical care was pretty good. The E.N.T. unit I had just visited was unusual in that most of the patients were beyond hope.

"You're wondering just exactly how much surgery you'll be doing — right?" Ted asked.

"That's what I'm here for," I said.

"Ninety-five percent of the head and neck tumor patients haven't a chance," he said bluntly. "So face it. The other five percent — well, I'll throw as much your way as I can." His shoulders slumped and his tone held more regret than flippancy. "A lot of cases pass through — we have a pretty high turnover."

I got back to specifics. While I was touring the wards, I had come across one case that seemed operable.

"Ted," I said, "what about Mr. Seth Rodeston?"

Dr. Bentley nodded. "He was admitted yesterday. Fifty-six years old, previous history of a carcinoma in the floor of the mouth just behind the chin, which was removed. Tumor has recurred in the jawbone. Probably operable. Maybe curable. Worth a try." I'm not sure why I was surprised that Dr. Bentley was so knowledgeable and obviously on top of the cases in his service. I would later discover that he was a tremendously efficient and dedicated man. "I'll meet you in the ward for four o'clock rounds," he said, "and we'll discuss it then."

As he rose to leave, a young red-haired doctor carrying a tray squeezed past. Ted Bentley's greeting stopped him.

"Jack, this is Dr. Moynihan. He's temporarily joining our Service. Don, this is Dr. Faber of Internal Medicine." With that and a wave, Ted Bentley disappeared.

Dr. Faber grinned and joined me at the table. "First day?"

"Yep."

"Met Anderson yet?"

"I've met him."

Jack shrugged. "He isn't the greatest, but . . ." He began shoveling in food. "Just don't take any shit from him." He looked out the window, and following his gaze, I noticed that the previously clear sky was becoming opaque, with ominous dark clouds moving in from the west.

"Must be a storm front coming in," Jack said. He shook his head. "God, I hope it doesn't rain!"

"You live in a flash flood area?"

He looked up, surprised. "No." Then he laughed. "Oh, you mean about the rain." He glanced outside again. "Like Ted said, I'm on the Medical Service.

Our wards are crammed already. Christ, we've got beds in the halls, in the reception areas, even in the conference rooms. If it rains, I don't know where in the hell we'll put them."

I tried to make sense out of his comments. Then he went on.

"Look, this is a government hospital, and any ex-serviceman who says he's sick is entitled to treatment. When it's cold and rainy, this is a great place to get a clean bed and three squares a day. Our caseload will go up about twenty percent."

"You don't have any control over admissions?" I asked.

"Very little. And damned little over discharges, either. You know, some of our patients are as good at avoiding getting out as they are getting in. When it's discharge time, they fake a heart attack — develop chest pain, complain of shortness of breath. They're experts. They know as much about symptoms as I do. Hell, I've got one patient who manages to *accidentally* fall out of bed every time I sign his discharge order. Last time, he really got a minor concussion. It made his day."

"Maybe he just doesn't have anyplace else to go."

"He hasn't. So what the hell; we let him stay. Actually, we're up to our asses in 'disposal problems.' Most of them could get along with outpatient care. But they haven't any money or families. So we admit them. And we keep them. A lot of them we keep until they die."

I realized I was in an alien world, and the first order of business was to get oriented. Right after lunch, I got on with it. Top priority was introducing myself to the Surgical Supervisor and staff, and inspecting the operating suites. Everyone was friendly, glad of extra help, and, from what I could discern, extremely efficient. The surgical rooms were beautifully equipped and perfectly maintained. Wandering through the diagnostic center, I was impressed by the very latest, most expensive and sophisticated devices, and the expertise of those functioning in that department.

I was feeling more relaxed about the entire situation. After getting lost only twice, I found my way back to the E.N.T. ward. Jeannette McGrory, the charge nurse whom I'd met earlier, went out of her way to be helpful. She explained the protocol, the routine, and the dozens of different forms which had to be filled out for services that, at University Hospital, could be accomplished in an instant by a phone call or jotting an order on a chart.

I was anxious to get to know the patients in the ward but, realizing it was the height of the afternoon, I decided to wait until after visiting hours. It was an unnecessary courtesy.

The scarcity of visitors was appalling. In other hospitals, the hours between two and four found the premises teeming with outsiders, anxious to see their loved ones. Yet only two or three visitors filtered into the ward. Each time the door opened, eyes from every bed looked up expectantly.

I continued with my appointed task of becoming as familiar as possible with the ward patients' histories and condition, while Mrs. McGrory filled me in on any points she might have overlooked.

"The main thing to remember," she said, "is that except for a few doctors and nurses, and a skeleton staff in Admitting, everyone works an eight-to-five shift. You have to plan accordingly."

Immersed in the charts, I nodded automatically. I hadn't quite finished when Dr. Bentley and Dr. Anderson arrived to begin rounds.

We went from bed to bed. Dr. Bentley seemed to have extraordinary rapport with the patients. His concern was genuine, and he had a small joke or a word of encouragement for each of his charges. Dr. Anderson was something else again. When an occasional patient voiced a complaint, the junior resident seemed to regard it as a personal insult, an affront to be argued and vindicated. I was liking him less and less.

We delayed seeing Mr. Rodeston until last, and when Dr. Bentley told him we were considering surgery, he became the center of attention. Every ear in the room was cocked to hear the details of hope. There wasn't a man in the ward who wouldn't have changed places with him.

I explained that the surgery we were proposing was complicated, and went into detail. It involved removing part of the jawbone and some of the tissue and muscles around it. That would, we hoped, get rid of the tumor, but we would then have to replace that tissue from an area outside the mouth in order to close the wound. I planned to create a flap by lifting all the skin from the forehead, leaving it attached only at one end in the temple area. A slit would be made behind the cheekbone and the flap would be threaded from outside into the mouth, so it could be stitched in place where the diseased tissue had been removed. A skin graft from his thigh would repair his forehead. I wanted to be sure Mr. Rodeston understood the magnitude of the proposed surgery, and I took a pencil and sketched out, as best I could, the entire procedure.

He gazed at my drawing. "It's like being scalped, isn't it? Scalped by an Indian."

I couldn't have put it better. There was no doubt that what I planned was mutilative surgery, but it was the only chance of saving his life.

"Well," I asked, once I was sure that he thoroughly understood, "I guess it's your decision."

"What decision?" Mr. Rodeston said. "I don't want to die, so go ahead."

"I can't promise a cure. All we can do is try."

He hesitated. The room suddenly erupted with opinions. It was like a television game show, with a portion of the audience urging the contestant to gamble with Fate; others cautioning him to stand pat. Anderson bristled. Bentley smiled. I waited.

I waited for what seemed a long time. "If you'd like to think about it — talk it over with someone," I suggested.

"I got nobody, doc," he said. "If it was your Pop, would it be go or no-go?"

I closed my eyes, picturing my father. The youngest

judge ever to sit on the bench in a Massachusetts court. Nationally prominent as a legal scholar, and for trying the "Boston Strangler" case. Strong, healthy, at the height of his earning power; nevertheless several years older than Mr. Rodeston. Surrounded by a loving wife and family. Vibrant, vital —

Lucky.

"I'd tell him to take a chance," I said.

"Good enough," Mr. Rodeston agreed. "The sooner the better."

"Tomorrow," I assured him.

I would need the usual preoperative tests — blood workup, X-rays, and all the rest. In a gesture to prove that I was "one of the boys," I drew the blood myself and requested that Mrs. McGrory get it downstairs for analysis as soon as possible.

Impulsively I picked up the phone, found the extension for the lab and dialed the number. A technician answered.

"This is Dr. Moynihan from the Head and Neck ward. I'm sending down a blood sample for a Mr. Seth Rodeston, who's scheduled for surgery tomorrow. Will you . . ."

The flat voice interrupted me. "It's ten till five."

"I realize that," I explained in my most ingratiating manner, "but this is important. I'd really appreciate your help. I'd like the results tonight and . . ."

I heard his words just before the phone went dead. "Fuck off, doc."

Chapter Fourteen

W ELL, THAT REMARK pretty well summed up the next three months. I discovered that because of his salaried position, a physician in a Veterans' Administration Hospital had little more clout, control, or status than the lowliest cog in the wheel. What the doctor did have was a helluva lot more responsibility. There were so many men to take care of.

Men. Oddly enough, during the entire time I was there, I never saw a female patient in the VA Hospital. It surprised me. Certainly there were former WACs and WAVEs eligible for admission, and I once asked Dr. Bentley about it. He shook his head, equally puzzled, and couldn't come up with a reason. Admittedly, most of the women who had joined the military forces during the war were, on the average, good-looking, aggressive, and intelligent. Maybe they'd made it into economic brackets that permitted private medical facilities.

Getting back to my immediate problems, for the

convenience of the lab, I wound up delaying the jaw-bone surgery on Mr. Rodeston an extra day. It went well, but only time would determine if we'd been able to bring about a complete cure.

After that, I learned how to be an intern all over again. Dr. Bentley was a rock and really cared about every case, but he was sunk in a morass of administrative detail and paperwork. Anderson, I discovered, was a professional goof-off — a "ghost," as the nurses and interns call a doctor who can never be located. Wherever the hell Anderson hid, he ignored the page. There were times, after a crisis when we would have sold our souls for an extra pair of hands, that I physically went searching for him. His car was there. It was empty. I inspected the lounges, the bathrooms, the cafeteria, and even began a paranoid peering behind unoccupied desks and into empty public telephone booths. When he eventually sauntered in, and I challenged him, his reply was always the same.

"I was at a meeting. What's the matter? Can't you handle it? If you have any complaints, buddy, just fill out form 5112/7A."

Before long, I didn't have the time or the energy to argue. We were so damned short-handed. There were never enough nurses and orderlies, and I ended up doing a great deal of the scut work. Especially at night and on weekends. The laboratory technicians, as I had pointedly been reminded, worked from eight to five, Monday through Friday. So did the clerks and other supportive personnel.

We had a *sick* group in our care, men with multiple problems and complications. Unlike patients on most wards, the majority were not getting better — they were getting worse. Hardly an evening or a weekend went by that potentially dangerous and unexpected problems didn't develop. I did urinalyses. I drew blood. I got specimens for bacteria cultures, and ended up taking them to the lab to do the gram stains myself. Invariably I wasted ten or fifteen minutes searching for the culture medium plates, and additional agonizing time checking and double-checking my findings. I had been taught lab techniques in medical school and during my internship, but the passing years had left me rusty and unsure. But it's amazing what you can do when there's no choice. I even learned to type rapidly with two fingers, for there were no secretaries available during the weekends or evenings. Requisition slips, labels, envelopes, and letters were pecked out by my suddenly clumsy fingers on a bright and shiny electric typewriter that had been meticulously covered by an equally bright and shiny girl until she next reported for her forty-hour week.

I remember one weekend when I was on call. I got to my apartment at two-thirty in the morning and was back at the hospital by six. The next day I ran my tail off and wound up spending most of the night with an acutely ill ex-marine who'd been transferred from the ward to the Intensive Care Unit. Because the patient was so sick, I decided to sleep in the hospital. Unfortunately, there were no facilities for the "on-call" doctor, so I curled up on an examining table in an adjoining office. After that wonderful night, I got up and dashed about the entire next day, holding my head at an odd angle to protect an aching neck and shoulder.

I guess I wouldn't have minded the general ward duties if I had drawn the amount of surgery originally anticipated, but, as Bentley had warned, while we had a lot of head and neck tumors, most of the patients had delayed too long in seeking treatment. Nine out of ten didn't have a snowball's chance in hell.

However, it wasn't completely unproductive. I vividly remember a number of incidents, small triumphs that counterbalanced the many disappointments and frustrations.

One was Morris Baedecker. He'd been transferred from a local hospital after a private surgeon had performed a radical operation to remove a tumor of the esophagus. A stoma, an opening, had been created at the base of his neck so he could be fed by a Levine tube. He had not tolerated these tube feedings well, partly because some years before he'd had ulcer surgery, and a large portion of his stomach had been removed. Following the tumor operation, he'd been in a private hospital until his insurance coverage had run out. Professional maintenance was mandatory; his wife was at her wits' end; and since the patient had served three years in the U.S. Navy, he was entitled to our services.

We examined him upon admission. Morris was five feet, nine inches tall — and weighed *eighty-eight pounds.* His cancer had extracted nutrients at a rapid pace before it was detected and removed, and necessary treatment by chemotherapy and radiation had compounded his problem by causing nausea, diarrhea, and even more drastic weight loss. Only a limited amount of malnutrition can be tolerated by the human body before death results. Unless we embarked on a crash program, Mrs. Baedecker would be wearing black within days.

What made the case even more pathetic — and challenging — was the fact that both Dr. Bentley and I agreed that reconstructive surgery on the esophagus was possible, but it was inconceivable in the patient's present state. Mr. Baedeker was one of the rare ones. With a lot of luck, he had a chance. The Senior Resident and I came to the same decision almost simultaneously.

"Let's try hyperalimentation."

Only a few years before, a team of researchers had developed a technique for successfully replenishing the nutrition of some debilitated patients. It involved injection of fluids with a high concentration of glucose — twenty percent instead of the five percent in the normal IV — along with amino acids, the essential component of protein. For many years, some specialists believed that if you fed a cancer patient, you would accelerate the growth of the tumor. This was proven untrue. Both Bentley and I were aware that hyperalimentation was being used not only in treating curable patients, but also in making terminal victims stronger and more comfortable in their final days. It was not without hazard, however, and we explained our proposed treatment plan to Morris Baedecker in detail. He was so demoralized, so weak, and he missed his wife so much, he would have consented to anything.

We inserted a catheter into the large subclavian vein under the patient's collarbone, for only a vein of that size could tolerate the substantial amounts of sugar. Then we began delivering at least four bottles of hyperalimentation fluid over a twenty-four-hour period. Mr. Baedecker was now getting over four thousand calories a day.

At first, nothing happened. Mr. Baedecker's weight didn't change. To ward off discouragement, Ted and I constantly reminded each other, and the patient, that his metabolism must switch from a negative to a positive state. And then, happy day! Mr. Baedecker began to gain weight. The pounds went on slowly at first, and then more rapidly. At the end of two weeks, he had gained seven pounds.

One day, about four weeks after we'd started the hyperalimentation, I was checking Mr. Baedecker's physical condition. The scales showed an increase of twenty-two pounds, and his muscles were already beginning to put on bulk, his skin tone was returning, and he was noticeably happier, stronger, and more active. I was jubilantly noting my findings on his chart when I was aware of a commotion in the corridor beyond. At the same moment, one of the floor nurses appeared at the doorway to the ward.

"Mr. Duggan's had an arrest," she shouted.

For a change, Dr. Anderson was nearby, attending a

patient — and we both responded automatically, pounding down the hall and into Mr. Duggan's private room at a dead run. Two doctors from another service, who'd happened to be passing by when the crisis occurred, were already working on him. Their terse reports as they continued their feverish lifesaving attempts, filled us in. Mr. Duggan had been eating his lunch when a piece of stewed chicken had lodged in his throat, blocking off the airway. Medically, he was in what is known as respiratory arrest — his breathing had stopped, but his heart was still beating — erratic, weak, but nevertheless beating. The doctors had managed to remove the chunk of food, had inserted an endotracheal tube, and were supplying oxygen by means of a respirator. With all their efforts, Mr. Duggan's blood pressure was very low, he was unresponsive to stimuli, and he was unable to breathe on his own.

Within the hospital's hierarchy, Dr. Anderson was the senior physician in the room, and as he watched the frantic efforts, his lips tightened, and he glared at the duty nurse.

"What in the hell's going on?" he snarled. "Can't anybody in this goddamned hospital read?"

I knew he was referring to a prominent notation on Mr. Duggan's nursing card, written there at his direction.

Almost everyone is aware of the official hospital charts kept on every patient, which are legal and permanent records. However, the uninitiated may not know that the nursing staff maintains a separate, temporary Kardex system, which condenses the physician's orders and prevents constant and time-wasting reference to the more voluminous charts. The necessary information is transferred to preprinted five-by-seven forms. In addition to the patient's name and bed number, there are perhaps half a dozen time-saving headings, beneath which are multiple-choice notations prefaced by a little box in which a checkmark can be placed.

For instance, one heading is *Activity*. The choices to be marked are "bedrest," "chair," "ambulate," "dangle," "commode," "ward privileges" — and "needs assistance." A single check in the appropriate box prevents errors and is a time-saving device.

Under *Hygiene* is "bed bath," "shower," "tub" — and so on. There is a much larger box on the card headed *Special Comments*.

It's a good system. All notations and checks are made in pencil, so that as the patient improves or deteriorates, orders can be changed by applying an eraser and making a new check. That same eraser can eliminate jotted notes based on oral instructions from the physician or personal comments by the nursing staff that might be embarrassing or a legal liability if made part of the official records. While policies differ in hospitals, usually the card is destroyed when the patient is discharged or dies.

I was well aware that under *Special Comments* on Mr. Duggan's card was a large notation: "D.N.R."

Do Not Resuscitate.

I had no quarrel with Anderson's order. Mr. Eugene Duggan was a World War I veteran, seventy-six years old, riddled with incurable cancer and beset with constant, agonizing pain. Dr. Anderson's directive meant that in case of a crisis, no attempt was to be made to save him.

There has been a lot of publicity lately about physicians withholding lifesaving techniques from terminal patients. A recent court case decided that a doctor who withheld available treatment was criminally liable. Yet I doubt if any practicing physician in the world has not searched his soul when artificially prolonging a hopeless case. Most doctors draw the line at actual euthanasia — or administering a drug that will induce death. But many have slipped into the room of a comatose patient who was being kept alive by outlandish scientific devices and quietly turned off a respirator or disconnected an IV. Such actions were never taken until every shred of hope was gone. No one on earth values life more dearly than the physician. When such an event occurs, other members of the staff cover for the doctor without comment, being in complete agreement with his merciful action.

But in Mr. Duggan's case, right or wrong, the resuscitation attempt had been launched. The doctors and nurse looked to Dr. Anderson for further instructions. It was his decision whether Mr. Duggan should be transferred to the Intensive Care Unit, or whether efforts should be discontinued, allowing the patient to lapse into death with dignity. It was a weighty decision.

"Jesus," Anderson whispered, half to himself, half to

me, "there's no way this guy can live out the week —
and everybody in this room knows it. If I order him to
the I.C.U., he's going to take up a bed — a bed that we
can use to save somebody who has a chance." He
thought a long time. No one commented. A life — any
life — deserved careful consideration.

"Disconnect the respirator," Anderson finally ordered. As soon as that was accomplished, every eye
went to the portable cardiograph monitoring the patient's heartbeat. All of us expected the feeble, un-
dulating line to falter and straighten, indicating death.
About a minute and a half went by, and then suddenly
Mr. Duggan began to breathe by himself. A few moments later, his heart settled into an almost normal
rhythm. His vital functions were returning. It was not
Mr. Duggan's day to go. With a little assistance from
drugs, his blood pressure returned to a satisfactory
level, and within a couple of hours, he came out of his
coma and was quite alert.

I would like to say that the experience caused me to
change my mind about doctors playing God. I would
like to say that I finally saw a trace of merit in the
recent court decision that life must be sustained, regardless of the circumstances. I would like to say that
the incident convinced me that "pulling the plug" was
unthinkable under any and all circumstances. I'd like
to say all those things, but I can't. Mr. Duggan died
less than a week later from the cancer that was sys-
tematically destroying one organ after another. I can
still remember his screams of pain, his begging for re-

273

lief. His was a slow, degrading death. Dr. Anderson's way would have been better.

As I've said before, the cosmetic field is mainly "happy surgery." At the VA, hopelessness and depression were a constant physical presence.

I don't know what I would have done without Patsy. Usually I was so beat and dead tired that the effort of driving all the way home seemed an insurmountable barrier, so Patsy loaded our son into the car on the Fridays preceding my weekends off and made the long trek to join me. Most of the time there was another passenger hitchhiking a ride. Marmalade, our Angora cat, usually rode along. Since she was an enthusiastic traveler, she often went for short jaunts around town with Patsy. But Marmalade was not used to all-day trips, and about halfway on their first visit, our cat became bored with counting the telephone poles whizzing past on the open road. The sun was beating in, and like any sensible feline, Marmalade decided to avail herself of some peace and shade, crawled under the seat for a siesta — and promptly got stuck! To the accompaniment of a yowling kitty and a crying baby awakened by the commotion, Patsy pulled over, got out and assessed the situation. Almost immediately, a Good Samaritan truck driver parked behind her, jumped out, and suspecting engine trouble, hurried up.

"Can I help you, lady?"

Patsy grinned. "You bet! How are you at extracting Angora cats from under car seats?"

Another time Patsy drove over alone. One of her sisters had been visiting and offered to babysit so Patsy and I could spend some time together.

It was an offer we couldn't refuse, and we excitedly made plans. We decided to take on Las Vegas and really do the town right. Neither of us had been there before, and in a burst of "cost-be-damned" enthusiasm, I reserved a hundred-dollar-a-night room at the most luxurious hotel and ordered a deluxe prix-fixe dinner.

Dressed to the teeth, we joined the crowd in the dining room — and then we both started to shake with silent laughter. Everywhere we looked were female breasts. See-through blouses, scanty halters, and necklines to the navel were favored by the lady diners. The waitresses were practically topless. To cap it off, there was a magnificently endowed female sommelier. Each time a male patron ordered a vintage wine, an added attraction was a neck massage, done with the customer's head cuddled between her ample breasts.

Even so, we hadn't realized the extent of the town's fixation until we were later wandering through the lobby arcade of chic boutiques. Nestled among them was a plastic surgery clinic that offered breast augmentation — with a sign proclaiming that the cost could be charged to one's hotel bill or to any national credit card.

But such diversions were few and far between. Those twelve weeks were mostly hellishly hard work, though during the three months I spent at the VA, I actually did fewer than a dozen operations. Still, it was more head and neck surgery than I would have drawn at University Hospital, and I was grateful for the experience. Besides, several cases with which I became involved resulted in great personal satisfaction.

Take Mr. Henry McNally. At the age of forty-two, Mac found himself well on the way to being a successful dairy farmer. Married, the father of two children, he had a herd of over forty prime Holstein cows, a couple of blue-ribbon bulls, a comfortable ranch house, a late-model car — and a very small lump on the left side of his face.

Every morning he felt the mass, kidded himself that it wasn't getting any larger — not much larger, anyway — and spent six more years hoping it would go away. On his forty-eighth birthday, the tumor was the size of a grapefruit, and a thick gauze pad was necessary to hide its chronic bleeding. Reluctantly renewing his acquaintance with the rural doctor who took care of his kids, Mac was referred to a surgeon, who diagnosed the mass as a huge hemangioma, a benign blood-vessel tumor. It was nonmalignant, but a major, life-threatening bleed was almost a certainty unless it was removed, and Mac had agreed to the operation.

The origin or cause of such a lesion is unknown, but its mass is composed of newly formed, intertwined spaghetti-like blood vessels, which constantly multiply. What early on would have been fairly uncomplicated surgery turned out to be extremely difficult because of the tremendous amount of bleeding and the considerable tissue involved. The tumor surgery had taken over ten hours, and twenty-two units of blood were needed. It had been a messy, taxing procedure, and a nerve was injured during the operation, causing paralysis of the left side of the face.

Although he'd promised to return for evaluation, Henry McNally turned in his membership card to the human race. Large amounts of cheap wine and dimly lit skid-row bars partially camouflaged his now deformed appearance. With all muscle tone on the left side of his face lost, Mac's cheek drooped until the nasal fold was erased. The corner of his mouth sagged, causing almost continuous drooling. When he sat in a bar, he was careful not to face a mirror.

Picked up on a common drunk charge, Mac was taken to County Jail, where a social worker urged him to seek voluntary admission to the VA Hospital.

We spent a week getting the alcohol out of his system, and once he was dried out, continued a regimen of nourishing meals and vitamins before scheduling him for surgery.

All three of us — Dr. Bentley, Dr. Anderson, and I — scrubbed in on the case. We'd come up with a two-phased plan, and since I had done a few facial paralysis cases, it was agreed that I should be the primary surgeon.

Our intention was to reopen the old incision and explore the area in hope of finding the main trunk of the damaged facial nerve and repair it. That was Phase One of our plan, but we admitted the odds were against success. It was our guess that, knowing that the tumor was benign, the original surgeon had not attempted to excise the entire hemangioma. To do so would have been terribly mutilative, necessitating the removal of almost the entire side of Mac's face. Locating that elusive nerve is difficult under the best of circumstances, and with the scar tissue from the previous operation, we knew that our hopes for repair were probably doomed. Nevertheless, it represented optimum results, and we spent almost an hour searching for that nerve trunk.

There was a significant amount of bleeding, but we were able to control it by using an electric cautery as a knife rather than the usual scalpel, coagulating the bleeders with the electric current as we incised. Once we got to where the facial nerve should be, there was a tremendous amount of scarring and a concentrated network of intermingled arteries that resembled a nest of tiny snakes. I wearily straightened.

"It was a good try, and we get A for effort — but we're kidding ourselves. Let's switch to Plan Two." Both Anderson and Bentley nodded their agreement.

We closed the original incision and made two others — one over the cheekbone and another at the corner of the mouth — and created a tunnel between the two. Then we took a piece of fascia, a tough, tendon-like tissue, from the patient's leg, and once it was trimmed to the appropriate size, slung it between the left cheekbone and the corner of the mouth. By cinching it up, we were able to pull the mouth to a position even with the other side.

I wished with all my heart that we could have offered Mr. McNally a repair of the nerve and a return of full function — but, that being impossible, we'd done the best we could. We had given our patient the gift of a neutral expression. It would allow him to have a relatively normal — though static — appearance. While it did not in any way solve the problem of the paralyzed muscles, we had effected a substantial cosmetic improvement. He need no longer be embarrassed to face the world.

I didn't realize how satisfied Mr. McNally was with our compromise until about two weeks later, when his face had nearly healed and the stitches were removed. I was passing by the public phone near the ward and heard him calling his wife. For the first time in many months, he informed her of his whereabouts. From what I could gather, their reunion promised to be a happy one. He hung up and looked at me, his eyes twinkling in an otherwise expressionless face.

"My family did the best they could with me gone, but it's been rough. I guess things at the ranch are in pretty bad shape. But we'll get by." He chuckled. "If vaudeville ever makes a comeback, I can always apply for a part-time job as straight man with a comedy team, right? And failing that, I'll bet I'd make a mint as a professional poker player."

Following the removal of his jawbone tumor, I saw Mr. Seth Rodeston every day. I was sure we'd gotten all of the malignancy, and his recovery went well. The flap that was threaded from his forehead into his mouth was temporary, and after the jaw was sufficiently padded, the unused portion of the flap was replaced on its original site. Actually, one third of his forehead required a skin graft. It was noticeable, but not too bad. From outside, the jaw looked normal. There was an unavoidable thickness inside his mouth that created a little difficulty. His speech was slightly slurred — but he could live with that. The important thing was that we'd cured his recurrent cancer.

There was a certain brand of humor always present amidst the grimness and morbidity of the cancer ward, and I suppose an outsider would label such flippancy unfeeling. But it isn't callousness that dictates the need for an occasional laugh; it's the necessity to ease the tension and retain perspective. I believe it was Mark Twain who wrote: "Everything human is pathetic. The secret source of Humor itself is not joy but sorrow. There is no humor in heaven."

At the VA Hospital there was pathos and sorrow — and since it sure as hell wasn't heaven, there was humor, too. I remember one Monday morning following a weekend off, when I asked Dr. Anderson how Mr. Rutledge was faring. Even I was a little shocked at his reply.

"The old gomer in bed eleven? He won't be around long. He's developed a positive O sign."

While I was trying to sort out the unfamiliar terms, Mrs. McGrory came to my rescue by explaining that "gomer" was a term often used to describe a particularly hapless type of patient — the one who habitually falls out of bed and accidentally overturns trays. The "O sign" was trade lingo to describe a patient lying in bed with his mouth open — like an O. The condition was usually present in those who were comatose and near the end of the road.

A similar description was the "positive Q" sign, denoting the same condition as described above, except that the patient's tongue was hanging out of his mouth, off to one side — hence the appearance of a Q. It had the same significance as "positive O," only more ominous.

But the macabre humor was not confined to the doctors, interns, and nurses. The patients contributed as well.

Mr. Edmund Budlow was a man in his late sixties who'd developed a cancer inside his mouth, behind his upper right molar. He had been reporting regularly as an outpatient for X-ray treatment, but the prescribed therapy had failed to control the tumor. It was now necessary to remove it surgically.

An hour or so after he was admitted, I sat beside him, taking his medical history. Even with age, he was a handsome, rakish man, and every time Mrs. McGrory or one of the nurses passed, he eyed her appreciatively.

"Have you ever had any venereal diseases — such as gonorrhea?" I asked. It was one of the standard questions.

"Jesus, boy," Mr. Budlow exploded with a guffaw. "Have I ever had it? Why, I'd be lonely without it!"

After making sure Mr. Budlow was joking and that

gonorrhea was not, at the moment, one of his problems, I outlined the major operation he was facing. To obtain satisfactory results, I explained, it would be necessary that we get every trace of the tumor. That meant massive tissue loss, removing half of the lower jawbone, and doing a radical neck dissection to excise the muscles and glands on the affected side. It was a deforming procedure.

"Hell, do anything you want above the shoulders," he said. "My face isn't the secret of my success. Just don't go removing anything below the belt."

We scheduled the surgery a few days later. It was an extremely tedious procedure and very challenging because of the number of important anatomical structures in the neck. One mistake — one slip — could cause a major problem. It took over eight hours. I did something during that operation that I'd never done before. Leaving our patient in the capable hands of the anesthesiologist and an assistant surgeon, we broke for a ten-minute lunch, ordering sandwiches and coffee sent up and going just outside the operating room to eat. It's very difficult getting through an extremely long operation without some nourishment, but that's exactly what most surgeons do. In some high-powered medical centers, such action would be considered sacrilegious. But I believe this thinking is shortsighted. I was exhausted and starving before the break. All of us had noticeably slowed down. Sure, we had to rescrub, but getting through the last two hours of the operation was a snap after that short recess.

Postoperatively, Mr. Budlow did extremely well, and one day I gave in to the urge to tell him about the luncheon incident. He laughed louder than anyone else in the ward.

"Hell, doc," he said, "why didn't you wake me? The least you could have done was invite me to join you."

It wasn't as weird as it sounded. His words reminded me of a British surgeon I'd met early in my career. He did many of his operations under local anesthesia. If an operation stretched past four P.M., everything came to a halt and tea was sent in, with the patient invited to enjoy the liquid refreshment, along with the surgical team.

Even the Lab and Radiology departments were not immune from black comedy. Everyone is aware of the connection between lung cancer and heavy smoking, but chronic smokers continue to puff. I was in the Radiology Department one morning when I encountered an envelope containing the chest X-rays of a newly admitted, three-pack-a-day patient whose film indicated cancer of the lung. Across the flap of the folder was a prominent scribble, probably written by the resident radiologist in a moment of frustration. It mimicked a well-known cigarette ad jingle: "Me and my tumor . . . we got a real good thing."

I spent the last day of my rotation at the Veterans' Administration Hospital winding up loose ends and saying good-bye to the staff and the patients. Medical school professors constantly caution against personal or emotional involvement, and that commandment is easy to keep in a private hospital, where patients are admitted, have their surgery, and are discharged within a week or so. But here, except for those who had died, and a pitifully small number who'd been cured and had someplace else to go, most of the men who were occupying beds in the wards when I arrived were still there.

During the three months, I had come to know them, and they knew me. They'd gotten into the habit of asking about my wife, following the growth and progress of my son, and vicariously sharing my weekend activities. I had become fond of them, sharing their war experiences, looking at family photographs, listening to their reminiscences of better times. I knew that Brian Murphy in bed eight was the current gin rummy champion, but that Johnny Phizer could beat him at checkers every time. I had admiringly examined the box of medals cherished by Wayne Sedacki in bed twenty-one. I had helped write personal letters, mailed them, and shared the agony of waiting for replies. They were like family. It was startling to realize that, with all the problems I'd encountered, I'd miss them. Damn, I'd miss them!

My last official medical act was examining Morris Baedecker, our hyperalimentation case. It had been seven weeks since we'd started treatment, and when Mr. Baedecker triumphantly stepped on the scales, the dial registered a hundred and twenty-eight pounds — forty pounds more than when he'd been admitted. His reconstructive surgery could be scheduled soon, and I felt a twinge knowing that I wouldn't be on hand to do it.

A few minutes later, Dr. Bentley and Dr. Anderson marched in, followed by Mrs. McGrory bearing a giant tray of homemade cookies, which she had baked the night before in honor of the occasion. In spite of the necessity for toothless and pain-ridden well-wishers to dunk the wafers in coffee or milk so they could be swallowed at all, the air of festivity was sincere.

The three months were over, and with a mixture of regret and relief, I went to collect my personal belongings — and to sign out for the last time.

Chapter Fifteen

THE MOMENT I ENTERED University Hospital, it was as if I'd never been gone. After three months at the VA, I was home again.

There were a few changes — and one of them was that the general surgery resident position on the Plastic Surgery Service was currently being filled by Dr. Isobel Waring.

I was in my office at the Outpatient Clinic, getting organized, when she popped in and extended her hand.

"Hi. Dr. Parmenter told me you'd be back today. He'd probably never admit it, but he's missed you. I'm Isobel Waring, M.D. — ready, willing, and able to learn."

She had a nice smile, and was extremely attractive. Tall, willowy, with light brown hair and green eyes — utterly feminine. I glanced at the clock: eight forty-five.

"Sit down," I said. "We've got time for a cup of coffee."

"Great." She took a chair. "You get the java, okay?" Her eyes twinkled. "I might as well tell you right off. I'm not exactly into the Women's Movement, but every time there's a gathering of doctors, I get pretty sick of being expected to fetch the coffee — just because I'm a female."

I grinned and returned with two steaming cups. "Fair enough, *doctor*. You won't have any trouble with me." We appraised each other for a few moments. "Have you decided on your specialty?" I asked.

"You bet. General surgery."

I nodded and took a deep swallow of coffee, and noticed her gaze was still glued on me.

"Well?" she asked.

"Well ... what?"

"Aren't you going to ask why a nice girl like me wants to be a general surgeon? Aren't you going to hint that it's a man's field — that the competition is too tough? That I'd be better off going into practice as a pediatrician or maybe a gynecologist?"

"The thought never entered my mind," I lied. There was silence. "But what's wrong with gynecology? Women doctors make it big in that specialty. Many patients feel more comfortable with a female gynecologist."

"I'll tell you what's wrong," she said. "I *like* general surgery — and I'm good at it."

"I didn't say you weren't. But you seem pretty uptight. Some of the male chauvinists around here giving you trouble?"

She frowned. "Nothing that I can't handle. Let's just say I'm a little tired of the gynecologist jokes. You know — 'I'm dilated to meet you' and 'If I can be of any cervix to you, let me know.'" She smiled, but her eyes were cold and determined. "And I'm sure you've heard members of that specialty referred to as 'spreaders of old wives' tails.' Sorry, it's just not for me."

She crossed her legs, and it was all I could do to keep my glance from her attractive knees. She noticed.

"Go ahead and look, doctor. I may be a physician, but I'm still a woman. Oh, and I ought to be honest — I'm not especially interested in the field of plastic surgery, but I've got a brain like a sponge. I'll listen and learn. I'll pull my own weight while I'm on this service."

"I'm convinced," I laughed. "We'll get along fine."

"Good," she said, taking my empty mug. "And since you brought the coffee, I'll rinse the cups."

I waited until she was almost out the door.

"Isobel . . ." She turned inquiringly. "As I said, I've got nothing against women surgeons." I paused for effect. "I just wouldn't want my sister to marry one."

I could hear her laughing as she went down the hall.

It was a little ironic that the first case I drew was very similar to one I'd seen just before my rotation at the VA Hospital.

Rulan Lee's parents had been born in a remote

Asian province and had emigrated, ending up in the United States, where their daughter was born. Miss Lee was quick to point out to me that she was a citizen; she wanted to be American to the core. Yet the only men she attracted were Orientals. She had nothing against them, she confessed, but she had little in common with them, either. She was determined to marry outside her own race — preferably a nice Southern California businessman. Miss Lee and her family lived just two doors away from Mrs. Muncie, the beautiful young Korean woman who had requested that her nose and eyes be made more "Caucasian" to satisfy her husband's desires. That procedure had been done by Dr. Parmenter and Dr. Burke while I'd been at the VA Hospital, and it had obviously been a rousing success. Admiring her friend's new appearance, Miss Lee decided to bring her problem to University Hospital, too.

There was one important difference. There are two types of Mongoloid features. Mrs. Muncie's had been typical of one — a tendency toward aquilinity, a rather oval face — and the nasal implant for the desired change had not been much of a problem. Miss Lee, on the other hand, had the other type — with the very flat and extremely broad nose found, for example, in many Japanese, Eskimos, and some tribes of American Indians.

I examined her face carefully. We had been able to use a preformed silicone nose implant for Mrs. Muncie, but none of the available sizes was exactly right to

give optimum results in Miss Lee's case. Our pros-
thetics department would have to come up with a
custom-made device for the bridge of her nose.

To accomplish this, a facial moulage would have to
be made. This is, essentially, a "life mask." The procedure is simple enough, but with a patient who is
even slightly claustrophobic or fearful, it can be an
uncomfortable experience.

With Miss Lee lying flat, a straw in her mouth as the
only air supply, we began applying layer after layer of
a compound çalled Alginate, an impression material
that takes approximately five minutes to solidify. Except for the area around the straw, every square inch of
the patient's face is covered with this congealing
material. Physiologically, there is no question that the
straw provides ample ventilation for breathing, but it
is easy to acquire a feeling of terror and impending
suffocation during the procedure.

Dr. Isobel Waring assisted, and we kept a steady
stream of conversation going. I knew from experience
that since the patient could not see, we had to reassure
her that we were with her every moment. Once the
facial moulage had dried, we carefully removed it in
one piece. It was sent to our prosthesis department,
where plaster was poured into the mold, producing an
exact replica of Miss Lee's face. From this, we experi-
mented to arrive at the most perfect nasal profile, and
then constructed an implant that would achieve it.

The surgery went well, and we were able to insert
the fairly sizable artificial bridge through an incision

inside the nostril. Then, with very fine wire, the prosthesis was stabilized so it could not rock or slip.

"Well, barring complications or a freak accident, that should do it," I said to Dr. Waring as we left the surgical suite.

She glanced at me, surprised. "What's this about freak accidents?"

I shrugged. "One of the first rhinoplasties I did was on a nineteen-year-old kid. I was pretty proud of myself. I had made him one very fine nose. Then, shortly after the surgery, our boy got to feeling independent and decided he could go to the john without help, so he didn't bother to ring for a nurse. Once in the bathroom, he flicked on the light and spotted himself in the mirror. Naturally, his nose was very swollen and splinted, and his eyes were black and blue. He took one look and promptly passed out. When he fell, guess what part of his anatomy hit the sink? The splint broke in two, but luckily my masterpiece wasn't damaged."

I grinned, remembering, and went on. "Then there was another rhinoplasty case I did. Everything was fine, and I gave the patient the standard discharge lecture about being careful. A few days later, he came into my office with his nose mashed to one side. He'd been in a minor automobile accident. Not another scratch on him — but he'd hit the dashboard and his nose took the brunt of it. Jesus, how come he didn't bump his arm or his shoulder . . . or even his butt?"

Dr. Waring thought for a moment. "I guess it's kind

of like — well, you know — nobody ever seems to slap you on the back unless you've got a sunburn. Maybe it's a version of Murphy's Law. If there's vulnerability, Fate will find it."

A minor surgical procedure scheduled a few days later seemed to lend credibility to Dr. Waring's theory.

It was one of those rare cases that are a snafu from start to finish. Joleyne Jennings was an extremely attractive young lady who was determined to break into television. She was, however, very concerned about a tiny cyst on the underside of her chin. Dr. Parmenter had seen her originally, and she had expressed irritation at a general practitioner from another hospital who had made an incision in the area and, after exploring, had insisted that the cyst didn't exist. Joleyne was terrified at the possibility of any disfigurement. She came into our Plastic Surgery Department with specific instructions — the cyst was to be removed, and any damage the G.P. had done was to be repaired, leaving an absolutely minimal scar.

It was a reasonable request. The first problem developed from a communication gap. Parmenter was scheduled to do the procedure with Dr. Waring assisting. At the last moment, he received an emergency call, so he told Dr. Waring she'd be doing the case with me. I got the message about the change in schedule, but was in my office making a phone call to a consultant. Dr. Waring assumed I'd be there within moments and she injected the Novocain to save time. Minutes passed, and I got a reminder call from Dr. Waring on the other line. Hurriedly putting my consultant on hold, I told her to go ahead — meaning that she should inject the anesthesia, which I had no way of knowing she'd already done. At any rate, when I got into the room, Dr. Waring had made a small incision and was fishing around in the tissue below the skin, vainly trying to locate the cyst. I hadn't had a chance to examine Miss Jennings's chin; in fact, I'd never seen her before in my life. Two strange faces working over her, when she'd expected Dr. Parmenter, did nothing for the patient's peace of mind.

"I can't find the darned thing," Isobel whispered, as I approached the table.

She'd done everything right; no one could fault her technique. I would have done the same. In a hurried, out-of-earshot conference, Dr. Waring admitted that the cyst had been perfectly obvious to touch before she'd started, but it had disappeared after the injection of the local anesthetic.

So we had an extremely vain and ambitious young woman whose biggest nightmare was ending up with a scar on her chin. And we had an incision — but couldn't locate the cyst. We fished around and fished around, but in spite of our efforts, we couldn't find it. I took out a little bit of fatty tissue beneath the skin, which might have been the offending lump, but we had our doubts. My feeling — my hope — was that the cyst had burst when the anesthetic had been injected; however, there was no way to be sure. Finally, defeated, we gave up and carefully closed the incision with a few very fine skin sutures.

The only open avenue at that point was complete

honesty. We explained to Miss Jennings what had happened, that we weren't sure whether or not the cyst was removed, that we would just have to wait and see if it redeveloped. To say that she was unhappy about the situation was the understatement of the year.

"You're both incompetent — and you're butchers," she announced coldly. "My attorney is Roger Fornsby. Remember the name. You'll be hearing from him!"

I had no doubt that we would.

Only that morning I had overheard two staff surgeons talking in the lounge.

"Hey, Joe," remarked the one, "remember when we were kids? How it was drummed into us that we would get rich when we grew up if we were honest, true, and worked hard?"

"Yeah," replied the other.

"Well, do you realize that's passé? The new American dream is to grow up and sue your doctor and get rich quick."

Joe grunted. "I saw a bumper sticker coming in this morning: 'Support your local attorney. Send a boy to medical school'!"

I have no intention of going into all the pros and cons of malpractice suits. Doctors are human, and occasionally mistakes are made and tragedies occur. In case of gross incompetence or neglect, I firmly believe that a patient is entitled to compensation. But those occasions are unusual. What most people fail to realize, I think, is that no physician can — or will — guarantee results. He can only promise his best effort. There is no expressed or implied contract with the patient that a cure will be forthcoming.

I also believe that the time has come to educate patients that they must share the risk with their doctors. A woman who waits a year after detecting a lump in her breast cannot present herself to her surgeon and demand that he cure her. The family who has watched a loved one chain-smoke for years has no right to seek legal recourse when lung surgery fails to save that life. The patient must not expect to hitch a totally free ride on another man's training, effort, and strength. Publicity has led patients to believe that men of medicine not only can — but must — work miracles. Realistically, the doctor stands ready with his skills, but they are limited. We try — we try like hell. It's all we can do.

It is my opinion that to save judicial time and taxpayers' money, a board must be established to separate legitimate complaints from the "crazies." Furthermore, I believe if an attorney convinces a client to sue on obviously ludicrous grounds and loses the case, the hospital, the insurance company, and the doctors involved should countersue the attorney for malpractice. They have a right to regain money spent in defending, for time, and for damages to reputation. With lawyers exposed to the same malpractice liability as the medical profession, the number of suits would be drastically cut.

There are other ways to avoid malpractice suits, too, and Dr. Parmenter demonstrated one technique. When Miss Jennings returned home, she phoned and demanded to speak directly with the Chief. As she vented her dissatisfaction, Dr. Parmenter listened patiently. Totally agreeing with every point and accusation she made, he concentrated on being sympathetic and solicitous. What she had gone through was inexcusable, he said. He made her promise to call him personally each week with a progress report. In the future, she could be assured that he would drop everything and attend her personally. Under his overwhelming charm, her anger evaporated. Apparently the needle had punctured the cyst, for it never recurred — and any legal retaliation planned by Miss Jennings was forgotten.

I settled into a comfortable, satisfying, day-to-day routine of dealing with my share of the numerous plastic surgery cases that were admitted. I was happy on the particular morning when I passed Miss Farrell's desk and she stopped me.

"Dr. Parmenter wants you in his office for a meeting at eleven A.M. sharp," she said.

Frequent consultations with the Chief of Plastic Surgery weren't unusual, but it was already ten forty-five. Pretty short notice. I wouldn't have thought too much about it, but I heard Miss Farrell imparting the same terse message via the phone to Dr. Burke and to Evelyn Grady, the Director of Nursing Services.

On the dot, the three of us met at Parmenter's office door and went inside. He asked us to be seated and fiddled uncomfortably for a few moments with a letter opener. It was unlike Parmenter to be ill at ease.

"I'm going to need your help." Dr. Parmenter's voice was tight and strangely formal. He allowed his gaze to roam the room, momentarily resting on each of us. "I'm going to need the help and cooperation of all of you." A few moments passed as he fingered the file on the desk in front of him. *"We've got a very hot potato on our hands!"* And then, in a low voice, he went on to fill us in.

Afterward, I half-listened to the low-keyed argument being waged between Mrs. Grady and Dr. Parmenter. I was still thinking my own thoughts, weighing the ramifications of what we had just been told. Finally Evelyn Grady's strident voice brought me back to the immediate problem at hand.

"I'll tell you again — I don't *have* a private room available!" she said.

The Director of Nursing Services was perhaps fifty-five, and her cherubic face, salt-and-pepper hair, and granny glasses belied a hard-nosed, no-nonsense woman whose years of experience and efficiency had made her one of the top professionals at University Hospital. She was completely responsible for the admitting procedures, the training, recruiting, hiring, dismissing, and assigning of nurses. She was superb at her job and absolutely indispensable. She knew it — and was impervious to intimidation by arrogant Chiefs of Departments, egotistical physicians, unreasonable patients, infighting, and institution politics.

"Look," Parmenter said nervously, "the plane arrives at twelve fifty-five today. That means Rittinghouse will be checking in around two at the latest. We've *got* to come up with a private room!"

Mrs. Grady shrugged. "What do you want me to do? Throw out a patient so we can accommodate this Rittinghouse?"

"Then what do you suggest?" Parmenter snapped.

Mrs. Grady glanced briefly at the records in the folder she'd had the foresight to bring with her. I got the impression it was an idle gesture, that she knew every patient in every room by heart.

"We'll probably have a private room available late tomorrow. In the meantime . . ." She peered again at her admission register. "We have an opening in 312. The other bed is occupied by Frank Massingill and . . ."

"Frank Massingill!!" The name escaped the Chief of Plastic Surgery's throat in a strangled yelp. "My God!! If Mrs. Rittinghouse has to share a room, it will have to be in the women's ward!!"

The Director of Nursing stared at Parmenter for a long moment.

"Just because this Rittinghouse had a transsexual operation, that doesn't make him a female — not in my eyes."

"Jesus Christ, Grady," Parmenter groaned. I'd never heard him use profanity before in mixed company. "Our patient was married to Randolph Rittinghouse three months ago. *Married in church.* Even in the eyes of God, Mrs. Rittinghouse is a woman!"

"God doesn't run my department, I do," Evelyn said. She allowed her gaze to drop again to the folder on her lap. "Except for 312, there's another possibility — a four-bed room. The other patients" — she read them deliberately without raising her eyes — "are Carl Barnes, Alex Polasky, and Bernard Feiner."

Parmenter remained silent until her eyes were forced to meet his. He had obviously decided on another tack, for his voice was low, controlled, conversational.

"Our patient," he explained casually, "has long, blond, shoulder-length hair. She's had hormone treatments, followed by breast implants. Electrolysis has removed any remaining masculine body hair. She has a vagina — inadequate, I admit — but that's why she's coming here."

There was silence in the room as each of us pictured the effect of such a patient being assigned to the men's ward. Mrs. Grady was the first to capitulate. She shook her head, but she was beaten and knew it.

"All right. We'll put him — her? — it! — in 502. But all three of the female patients in that room are elderly, and I don't want any static from the floor. I must insist that the curtains around the Rittinghouse bed be kept closed at all times and . . ."

Parmenter nodded happily and interrupted. "And that brings us to the next order of business. Even though this will only be a corrective operation, I'm sure we're all agreed on the need for discretion. If the press got wind of this, I don't know whether or not they'd be interested, but . . ."

"They'd be interested, all right!" Mrs. Grady couldn't help interjecting.

"But," Parmenter blandly continued, "I don't want to take a chance that this place will be teeming with reporters. The patient will be merely listed as Mrs. Robbie Rittinghouse, and the surgery will be posted as a routine vaginoplasty."

Dr. Burke had been sitting quietly, uneasily. "How in the hell did we get roped into this?" he suddenly blurted. "There are hospitals that have gender identification centers that take sickie cases like this."

Burke had a point. Sex-change surgery should be done only in medical centers that have set up a special team of doctors to handle transsexual patients. There are several in the United States. Surgeons, psychiatrists, endocrinologists, and urologists work together on each case. Candidates are well screened. For a prospective patient to be eligible for consideration, the investigating board must be assured that the patient is a true transsexual, not a homosexual or lesbian. According to psychiatric terminology, a transsexual is a person who honestly believes he was born the wrong sex, one who is psychologically "a female in a male body" — or vice versa.

"We've never done any sex-change surgery before," Burke continued.

"And we don't intend to start doing it," Parmenter said. "But those centers are set up for patients *contemplating* such surgery. Mrs. Rittinghouse made her decision almost two years ago. She had the sex-change surgery done in Europe. They botched it, and she ended up with a two-inch-deep vagina. All we're doing is reconstructive surgery. It's a standard procedure.

Robbie is no different from any other female with a vaginal defect."

"The hell she isn't," Evelyn Grady and Albert Burke chorused.

"I'm still wondering how we got roped into this," Burke pressed.

Parmenter shrugged. "I guess you might say I goofed. Early this morning I got a call from a doctor in Berkeley. All he told me was that a friend of his had recently married and the couple was having difficulty during intercourse because the wife suffered from a vaginal anomaly. He asked if we could take her as a patient and I said we would. Then he dropped the bomb and gave me the details. I started to hedge, but this referring doctor's a pretty militant guy, a homosexual himself. He's burning because Rittinghouse has been kicked around by one surgeon after another. There's an attorney up there considering legal action — a class action suit on behalf of the entire gay community. He promised discretion if we took the case — and a stink like you couldn't believe if we refused."

Burke grunted. He saw the wisdom of Parmenter's decision, but like Evelyn Grady's, it was obvious that his sensibilities were offended by the entire situation. Parmenter was quick to see this, and glanced at me.

"Don," he said, "you're the only one who hasn't been turned off by the whole idea. Do you have any objection to taking primary responsibility? I'd be grateful if you could. Naturally, any problems, just let us know and we'll come running."

I glanced at the set faces of Grady and Burke. I had a mental image of how fast they'd move if I needed them. And when the chips were down, I knew that Parmenter had perfected the ability of walking through mud without getting his shoes dirty. I felt queasy, too. It was outside the norm, and I was struggling with a gut reaction. I wish I could say that the Hippocratic oath — by which I had sworn to provide, to the best of my ability, medical help to all who needed it — had something to do with my decision. But frankly I also felt it was one hell of a teaching case.

"Okay," I heard myself saying, "tell Admitting to let me know as soon as she arrives."

Instead of eating lunch, I headed for the library. Although University Hospital's collection of books and articles was huge, there was very little available on the subject of transsexuals. I was surprised that Grabb and Smith's *Plastic Surgery*, the acknowledged "cookbook" constantly referred to by our specialty, devoted a few paragraphs to vaginoplasties, but studiously ignored its application to transsexual operations.

I did discover that, surprisingly enough, the sex-change operation is being done in fewer institutions each year, even though the demand for them has increased. For instance, the procedure is no longer done in Denmark — the country that started it all in the 1950s with Christine Jorgensen. From what I could determine, one reason for this decline was problems with postoperative patients. In spite of thorough screening, many developed severe psychiatric difficulties. Some decided that they wanted to change back to their original sex, and flipped out after realizing it was impossible. A few suicides have occurred. Even the more satisfied patients seem to express an insatiable need for more feminizing surgery — such as pleading for uterus and ovary transplants so they might bear children. Again, impossible. Faced with such problems and the great amount of support and counseling required, psychiatrists began refusing cases, and reputable surgeons were reluctant to do the procedure without adequate psychological backup.

The page interrupted my research to inform me that Mrs. Rittinghouse had arrived, so I headed for her room. Pausing at the door, I nodded at the other three patients and noticed with relief that, as Mrs. Grady had decreed, the curtains completely shielded the occupant of the fourth bed. But before I could enter, the charge nurse hurried up and drew me out of hearing range.

"Well, it's already hit the fan," she said. "You know Mr. Dandridge, the son of the patient in bed three? He's demanding that his mother be moved. Says he's not going to have her sharing a room with — how did he put it? — that 'freak.' "

Before I could reply, the elderly Mrs. Dandridge, who was almost recovered from gallbladder surgery, came tiptoeing from the room.

"Did my son tell you I wanted my room changed?" she began in a timid whisper. The nurse nodded. "Well, forget it," Mrs. Dandridge said. "I'm staying where I am. It's about time something happened to liven things up around here."

The nurse rolled her eyes heavenward. With all our preplanning and caution, we had not taken into account that peculiarity found in every hospital — the "white underground," a grapevine that passes along news with unbelievable speed and accuracy. Within thirty minutes of Mrs. Rittinghouse's admittance, at least half of the staff and patients knew about her. Before the day was over, the families of the other two patients would make similar outraged complaints and demands, although the elderly ladies directly involved found Mrs. Rittinghouse fun and a good companion.

I don't know what I expected, but Mrs. Rittinghouse had been a big man — five feet, ten inches tall, and a hundred and eighty-four pounds. Naturally, surgery hadn't changed the brawny physique. The voice that returned my greeting was a low contralto, rather masculine, but as I approached, Mrs. Rittinghouse extended her hand in a completely feminine manner. I was fascinated by the size of her biceps and muscular forearm — a result of lifting heavy trays, for I would later learn that Mrs. Rittinghouse had worked as a busboy and waiter for three years to pay for the original surgery. The fingers of that large, square hand were tipped with the long, artificial sculptured nails available in expensive beauty salons. Her hair, as Parmenter had promised, was long and blond, and matched her arched and plucked eyebrows. Electrolysis had removed any sign of a beard, and her makeup was in good taste. The outlines of her breasts were visible

beneath the provocatively low cut yellow nylon garment she wore instead of the hospital gown.

I took her medical history. She was twenty-six years
old and had undergone the transsexual surgery about a
year and a half before. Six months later, after intensive
hormone therapy, she'd had her breasts done. Her replies to my questions were complete, straightforward,
polite, and occasionally touched with good-natured
humor. She was as anxious to put me at ease as I was to
gain her confidence.

In the course of my physical examination, I was surprised by the outdated technique that had been employed in Europe. The surgeon there had amputated
the penis and testicles, and after creating a pouchlike
space, had inverted the empty sac of scrotal skin to
form a vagina. But the scrotum is hair-bearing and the
skin available is limited, so the patient had ended up
with a shallow, fuzzy vagina that measured approximately two inches. A better operation is now available.
Before the penis is removed, its skin is carefully undermined and retained — and then utilized to construct a vagina of adequate size. Even as I was finishing
the examination, my mind was forming a plan for the
corrective surgery.

"Mrs. Rittinghouse," I told her, "right now there
are a few things I have to do, but I'd like to come back
after dinner to discuss your problem and the solution
in more detail."

"Thank you, Dr. Moynihan," she said. "You've been
very kind."

I had formulated a reconstructive technique that I

was sure would work. It involved entirely removing the short vagina of scrotal skin and replacing it with a new, longer one constructed from skin grafts taken from the patient's thighs. One problem would be to find something to use as a stent, a mold, around which the skin graft could be wrapped, inserted, and held in place after I'd created the space for the vagina. I wanted to have on hand both some hollow and solid tubes; I would decide which to use during the actual surgery.

I left the hospital early that day, and went to a large hardware store. I asked the salesman in the electrical department to cut me pieces of plastic pipe — the first to measure two by seven inches, and the second, one and a half by six and a half inches. Evidently he'd never had an order for such short lengths before.

"Are you sure those measurements are correct?" he asked in an effort to be helpful. "What kind of plumbing are you planning?"

"It's very specialized," I said, straight-faced.

From there I hurried to the nearby five-and-dime and purchased Styrofoam cylinders in three different circumferences. Next I went to a local drugstore and asked for three packages of condoms, requesting a receipt.

"I can take them as a tax deduction," I explained. I imagine the clerk's perplexed look would eventually be duplicated when an auditing IRS agent came across that little item.

After a quick dinner with Patsy, who enjoyed the

account of my shopping experiences, I drove back to the hospital. Crossing the lobby, I was hailed by one of the medical students. He was practically panting with interest.

"Hey, Dr. Moynihan. Can I see her? Can I just peek in?"

"No," I snapped, "stay the hell away from her room, understand?"

A bit crestfallen, he shrugged. "Gee, I just wanted to give her a book. Nothing wrong with that, is there?"

"What book?" I demanded suspiciously.

"You know, the one by that transsexual tennis player."

He paused for effect. "It's called," he snickered, *"Tennis without Balls!"*

I started to retort, and gave up. I had a feeling I'd better get used to the locker room humor that would be coming my way. Then a sobering thought struck. Mrs. Rittinghouse had lived with such remarks for a long time.

I don't know how it happened, but after I'd explained my approach to the surgery to Mrs. Rittinghouse, little by little she told me her life story.

Robert Gaines, destined to become Robbie Rittinghouse, was the youngest of five children born over a twelve-year span to Arthur and Dorothy Gaines, who resided in a middle-sized town in central Ohio.

Robbie confessed that at a very young age he knew in his heart that he was somehow "different." As he grew older, he began to have trouble in school. He found physical education classes unbearable — the rough-and-tumble contact, the group showers, the horseplay, the grab-assing — all of it repelled and terrified him. A sympathetic doctor wrote a letter excusing him from the required sports activities, and when the school authorities demanded that he choose an alternate subject to fill the gap, Robbie chose home economics.

While the entire community and his schoolmates suspected that he was homosexual, the Gaines family was well regarded and the town considered itself civilized. Except for an occasional epithet such as *sissy, fairy,* or *little fag* being hurled at him by the less tolerant, he encountered surprisingly little physical abuse or harassment.

Until he entered high school. For the record, Robbie was not a practicing homosexual. But neither was he attracted to girls. He was at that time, in his own words, "neutral." He shunned sex entirely. The drive wasn't there. Then, early in his junior year, he was the victim of an attempted gang rape. Terrified, he took off and ended up in Seattle, where he quickly got a job as a busboy at one of the better-known hotels.

Up until this time, Robbie had never been to bed with a woman. A young waitress, intrigued by his gentleness and good looks, invited him to her apartment and, with a sudden determination to find out what he'd been missing, he went. Midway through the preseduction romp, Robbie was forced to admit the truth. He was not turned on by the woman. He felt nothing for *any* woman! So as not to insult her, he'd lied to the girl. Unaware of the irony, he'd blurted that he had a headache — and fled.

He lived simply and was able to get along on his salary and tips very well. He even managed to save a fair amount each week.

I'd been listening intently as Robbie recounted her past, and I took advantage when she paused for breath.

"What made you decide on the transsexual operation?" I asked.

Robbie thought a long time. "I suddenly realized I was a woman! I don't give a damn if nature goofed. *I was a woman!!*" She became less emotional as she continued. "I started to hear about this transsexual operation. I gave it a lot of thought and began asking around. I knew I had to be careful. It's pretty tricky not to get taken."

"What do you mean?"

"Well, there are some doctors willing to make a fast buck by doing the surgery, but most of the hospitals won't let them. Then I heard about a private clinic — but I found out it was a real rip-off. They promise the operations, and the poor kids that get involved hustle the streets for years to come up with the five thousand dollars the clinic demands. They insist that the prospective patients pay a little at a time, and give them receipts. They dispense estrogen that's so low-grade that even veterinarians won't use it. That's their idea of hormone therapy. Then they start adding extras — and more extras. It never ends. Somehow, no matter how much the kid had paid, it's never quite enough. And the patients, they're desperate — but hell, they can't sue. They'd never win. Public opinion's against them."

A nurse came in to take my patient's temperature and pulse. I bristled when she took Robbie's wrist as if it were a boa constrictor, but I held my tongue. Our conversation continued after she'd left.

"Where were we?" Robbie asked. "Oh, yeah! Anyway, I decided to go a different route. I saved my money until I had enough, then headed for Europe and had the surgery. I was told that everything would be okay. Afterwards, I met Randy, my husband. We fell in love and got married, but . . ."

"Robbie, I know you're not a homosexual," I interrupted. "How come you got married in a gay church?"

She grimaced. "I don't know if you can believe this, doc. I hope I can make you understand. Randy and I are in love. We're the best thing that ever happened to each other. We wanted our marriage to be sacred. But the minute a justice of the peace or a minister glanced at my birth certificate, none of them would touch us with a ten-foot pole. One minister actually threw us out, saying we were defiling the house of God. At least the pastor in Berkeley understood our problem."

I thought of the clinical definitions that I had learned. *Homosexual:* one with desires directed to a person of the same sex. *Heterosexual:* one with natural sexual desires toward the opposite sex. *Bisexual:* having both active (male) and passive (female) sexual interests or characteristics. Robbie didn't fit into any of the standard groupings. And then I mentally castigated myself. Why did I have to fit my patient into a category? She was simply a human being with special needs that were so strong that she had been willing to endure harassment, mental anguish, and the pain of multiple operations — all to attain fulfillment of those needs. What right did anyone have to act as judge?

"I love my husband so much," Robbie whispered, "I want to please him, to satisfy him. It's going to be all right, isn't it?"

"I'll do my best."

Two days later, Robbie was scheduled for surgery. When I walked into the operating suite, the scrub nurse automatically asked me if I had any special instruments that I wanted her to have ready on the surgical table.

"Yes indeed," I said. "Six dildoes, eight condoms, and two plastic pipes." She was flabbergasted, and I still remember her dutifully unrolling each condom and laying them all in neat rows on the table.

I happened to glance toward the window at the side of the room near the scrub sink. No fewer than twelve faces were pressed up against the glass, peering in. The nurses and technicians in the O.R. had gotten wind of the case and were beside themselves with curiosity. This self-appointed audience dispersed only after I ordered the circulating nurse to tell them to beat it.

The operation itself consisted of excising the tissue lining the short existing vagina and then making a deeper, wider space. Before going any further, I tested my makeshift stents. It turned out that the Styrofoam cylinders wouldn't work because they were straight, and the vaginal space curved upward, so I opted for the plastic pipe. I generously lubricated it with Vaseline and rolled a condom onto it. Then skin grafts, taken from Robbie's inner thighs, were stitched around the phallus-like structure, with the grafts inside out so they would adhere to the wall of the tissue in the space created. The lubricant would enable us to slip the plastic pipe out once the graft was properly positioned. The mold was inserted into the vaginal space as far as it would go, and I inserted packing down the pipe, which pushed the grafts even deeper and held them firmly against the side walls. Then the piece of pipe was slowly withdrawn. A heavy pressure dressing was placed over the outside of the vagina to hold the pack in place.

Postoperatively, Robbie's recovery went well. Certain problems did develop, but of a nonmedical nature. My patient was well aware of the disdain with which many of the staff regarded her. But forty-eight hours after the surgery, she was feeling well enough to kid about it.

Strangely enough, my biggest ally was Miss Farrell. To her, a Parmenter patient was a Parmenter patient. She considered it part of her job to make sure they were happy, that they had no complaints, and that they were treated with respect. When a few of the snide remarks reached her, she appeared on the floor one morning. A few pointed words to the resident and charge nurse brought all open hostility to a halt. She had power and they knew it. As additional insurance, she waited until everyone would notice and dropped in to visit Mrs. Rittinghouse to make sure she was satisfied with the way everything was going.

On the tenth day after the surgery, Robbie was well enough to go home. Just before signing her discharge slip and saying good-bye, I'd been in the outpatient clinic, piercing the ears of a fourteen-year-old girl. Somehow those two actions seemed to epitomize the profession I'd chosen. In the course of a few minutes, I'd indulged a young girl's fancy for tiny golden hoops, and I'd been successful in changing the body, and certainly the life, of another human being. The name of the game was happiness.

Happiness! Everybody finds it in a different way.

For Mrs. Frederick Baynes, I guess it was having her reconstructed breasts resemble as closely as possible her natural ones.

Here was a woman whose troubles had started when she sought breast enlargement.

It seemed cruelly ironic that after all the reconstructive surgery, her breasts were approximately the same size as before the ill-fated silicone injections. But we had done the best we could under the circumstances.

During a final checkup, I was pleased that she looked reasonably good after the prosthesis implants and the areola grafts. But her new breasts lacked nipples, and she was willing to undergo one more additional surgical procedure to get them.

There are various ways of creating protruding nipple mounds, and Dr. Parmenter and I agreed on a course of action. It was comparatively simple. Under local anesthesia, we made an incision behind one ear and, with a punch graft, removed four discs from the ear cartilage. They were taken from slightly separated areas of what's called the concha, close to the canal. It's a procedure that creates no deformity at all. We repeated it on the other ear.

Four of the discs were laid one on top of the other, as if we were stacking poker chips, and two catgut stitches were taken to hold them in alignment. From a small incision at the side, we were able to create a little tunnel to the middle of the areola and make a pocket of sufficient size to accommodate the cartilage discs. We closed the incision and repeated the surgery on the other breast. Light dressings were all that was needed. It is true that the cartilage-constructed nipples would be firmer than normal nipples, which are pliable, but cartilage tends to soften as times goes by.

The result was more than satisfactory.

The next day, Dr. Burke and I were making rounds together and stopped in to see Mrs. Baynes. Except for some mild swelling, things couldn't have been better.

Our patient was in a double room, and the other bed was occupied by a woman scheduled for a minor operation. I noticed that Ronnie Cosgrove, who had just recently been assigned on a rotating basis to the general surgery service, was taking her case history. At any rate, just as Burke and I were leaving the room, Cosgrove's patient stopped us.

"Pardon me," she said. "Mrs. Baynes told me who you were and that you'd probably be coming in. She says you're the greatest. Do you have a minute?" We nodded. "I've been thinking about having a face-lift," she admitted, "but I can't make up my mind. What do you think?"

Burke took over, cocking his head and professionally studying her appearance. Her face had considerable wrinkling and sagging skin. Burke told her he thought a face-lift would make an appreciable difference. The woman vacillated, still unsure.

"You don't have to decide right now," Dr. Burke said. "Think about it. You can always reach us at the clinic."

Ronnie, having finished his workup, was right at our heels as we started out the door. Suddenly his patient called after us.

"Thank you, Dr. Burke. But you know — I think I'd like a second opinion."

Hardly missing a beat, and without turning, Ronnie shrugged. "Okay," he said, "you're ugly!"

Outside, Burke and I stood rooted, absolutely dumbfounded. We had no way of knowing whether Cosgrove's remark had reached the woman's ears. Burke stared at Ronnie. Unable to utter his outrage, he spun around and took off toward the Administrator's office.

I turned on Ronnie. "What's wrong with you?" I said. "Are you retarded or something? How in the hell could you . . ."

Cosgrove blinked. "What'd I do?" It actually took a few minutes before he recalled his words, and then he became beet-red, genuinely contrite.

"It just popped out," he admitted. He glanced at the room and then back at me. "Boy! I'd better get in there and apologize and . . ."

Now it was my turn to be confused. If the patient *had* heard the remark, all the "I'm sorrys" in the world wouldn't help. But if she hadn't heard . . .

"If I were you, I'd drop it," I said. "Just cool it, understand?"

Thank goodness, Ronnie's words hadn't reached the patient. He got off with a reprimand. Good doctors are hard to find, and Cosgrove had the skills and basic intelligence to be a fine one. Age would mellow him and impart the necessary social graces. We hoped.

Happiness, to me, was being a plastic surgeon — having the experience and knowledge that I could competently treat any case in my specialty — as well as or better than any other surgeon. It wasn't ego or conceit, it was self-confidence.

So many people had helped me earn my M.D. — my parents, who'd aided me financially, the professors who had taught me, all the authors who'd learned and had the dedication to reduce their findings to the printed word so that others might benefit from their experiences, and the countless nurses and technicians and administrators.

Way at the top of the list was my wife, Patsy, who'd

put up with my moods and crazy schedules. She was once again pregnant — two months along. And my son Trevor, the brightest and handsomest kid on the block, would be two years old in a couple of months. My joy was boundless.

Chapter Sixteen

THROUGH THE YEARS I had always tried to do the best for my patients medically. Over and above that, I'd prided myself on understanding their fears, on being sympathetic. Yet, thinking back on it, how could I have really known how they felt?

This was a problem that was soon to be rectified — but dear God — did it have to come about in such a frightening and horrible way?

"Why is he holding his arm like that? Did he twist it or something?" I asked.

Patsy's eyes followed my gaze as Trevor yanked the cord attached to an animated bear, his favorite toy, forcing it to follow him across the room. Chubby, lightly tanned, and with a mass of blond curly hair, our twenty-one-month-old son could have won a "baby beautiful" contest anywhere. But even as we watched, he again placed his arm over his lower right chest as if it were tender or painful.

"I don't know," my wife said. "He's been doing that

for a couple of days. Not all the time — just occasionally." She scooped him up and they headed for the fun-filled ritual of his nightly bath. I joined with them later in the nursery to say goodnight and to listen solemnly and comment on the bedtime story Patsy read him each night. She glanced at me.

"I just took his temperature." She handed me the thermometer. He was running a low-grade fever of 100 degrees. I wasn't especially alarmed. Still —

"Why don't you call the pediatrician in the morning?" I suggested. "A check-up wouldn't hurt."

Around ten A.M., Patsy called me at the office. "I'm at the pediatrician's," she said. "He thinks it might be pneumonia. They've ordered some tests."

"I'll meet you in the lab," I said.

After they had taken the films, Patsy and Trevor waited outside, but I hovered around the department. I saw the technician take Trevor's newly developed chest X-ray into a radiologist for viewing. He quickly glanced at it — peered more intently, and then, with a concerned look on his face, hurried to the Chief of Radiology so that both of them could analyze and read it together. Without waiting to be invited, I joined them.

The chest X-ray was abnormal! They weren't sure what it was — but there was absolutely no visualization of the lower two-thirds of our child's right lung. Either there was a huge mass in there — or Trevor had a bad case of pneumonia, with the infection accounting for what is technically called a "white-out."

Our pediatrician diagnosed the problem as pneumonia and put Trevor on a program of antibiotics. After a week, we took him back to be reevaluated. Another chest X-ray showed no change. He had not responded to the medication.

Now the gears went into motion. A complete workup was ordered to try to determine what the mass might be. Trevor had blood tests — nothing amiss there. He had scans, which indicated a normal liver. The thoracic surgeons, the chest specialists, were called in. At first they considered a bronchoscopy — looking down the trachea with a tube — but they finally decided it was a needless procedure. It would tell us nothing except that there was a mass in Trevor's chest — and that we already knew. The conclusion was that it must be removed surgically. An echogram was ordered, a test involving sound waves that is supposed to indicate the consistency or makeup of the abnormality. We had considered the possibility of a solid tumor, and it was what we feared most — but the presumptive diagnosis, based on the echogram, was a large, fluid-filled congenital thoracic cyst.

If I have not touched on Patsy's or my emotions during this short period, it is because we were *numb!* Numb with worry and fear and disbelief. The new findings, however, made us feel pretty good, because even though we didn't relish the thought of our baby undergoing major surgery, knowing that it was a benign, correctable problem — really not that uncommon — made it much easier.

Once we were home, I tried to ease the tension. Patsy *was* pregnant, and I was concerned for her.

"Honey, would you like to go out somewhere for a really great dinner?"

"You — you mean — get a babysitter?"

"I'll go get some take-out food," I said.

We both realized that neither of us could bear leaving Trevor for a moment.

But even though we were concerned, we weren't terribly worried. Both of us stayed in Trevor's hospital room the night before the operation, playing with him until he went to sleep. I was successful in convincing Patsy to remain at home the next morning. After all, I argued, Trevor would be sedated. I would be checking on him constantly until he was wheeled to surgery, and I would call her the instant the operation was over. And to guarantee my own equanimity, I had deliberately booked a minor case in the Plastic Surgery Clinic at precisely the time Trevor was scheduled for his operation in the main O.R.

I remember it all so vividly. I had taken the skin cancer off my female patient's upper lip and was doing a full-thickness graft to replace the tissue. I had routinely sent the specimen down to the Pathology Department for confirmation that I had gotten it all — and I was irritated by the length of time they took to get back to me.

Little did I know at that very moment those pathologists were examining a *seven-pound cancer removed from the chest of my twenty-three-pound son!!*

When my own case was finished, I went back to the office. I knew Trevor's surgery had started about nine A.M., and when it got to be a quarter of twelve, I began feeling twinges of concern. As I reached for the telephone, Miss Farrell called me on the intercom. Two doctors were on their way in.

Before I could reply — or even stand up — the door opened and Trevor's pediatrician and one of the consulting thoracic specialists entered. I knew neither had been involved in the actual operation, but they had been observing.

"I'm afraid we have bad news for you," one murmured.

His words were like a physical blow. I was stunned. Were they telling me my son was dead?

They quickly went on to let me know about the seven-pound malignancy. I was speechless.

I found myself banging my fist repeatedly on the desk.

"Oh, dear God, no!" I fought for breath.

The doctors were mouthing words. Something about the fact that from the anesthetic and surgical point of view, Trevor was doing well — that the operation would be completed shortly — that they were sorry about the disastrous biopsy report, rhabdomyosarcoma, and —

That brought me up short. Rhabdomyosarcoma — one of the most malignant types of cancer — and so large that it had collapsed the lower two lobes of Trevor's lung!

Then they left.

I sat in my office, staring at the wall, in a state of shock — fighting dizziness and nausea. And then I thought of Patsy. What if she called the hospital? I couldn't tell her the news over the phone. I couldn't!

Like some kind of wild man, I sprinted for my car. We lived twenty minutes away and I recall driving along the freeway in a frantic, half-dazed fashion. As I turned off at the exit ramp, I spotted a car coming onto the freeway going in the other direction — a red Pinto station wagon, the kind of car Patsy had. For a moment I thought it was Patsy on her way to the hospital — she would discover what had happened before I had a chance to tell her! Should I go back? But I couldn't be sure, so I raced the rest of the way home, and through blurry eyes saw that her red Pinto was still in the garage. I ran into the house.

Patsy looked up, startled. "You're — you're home. Is Trevor okay? Is it over?" Her eyes searched my face.

I took her in my arms and told her. She was stiff, stunned, unyielding. Then she put her head on my shoulder and cried. We both cried. It was terrible.

After a while we called the hospital and found out from the recovery room nurses that the operation was over and Trevor was doing well. We also talked with the surgeon, who confirmed everything we knew. He suggested we wait until evening to visit our son.

There wasn't anything we could to in the meantime. It may sound strange, but after vacantly wandering around for a while, we both decided to lie down and try to sleep, not because we were tired, but because sleep is an escape — a far safer escape than drugs or alcohol. If you can get to sleep, at least it allows you to escape briefly the tremendous burden, the horrible sadness. And it makes the time pass.

When we walked into the recovery room, Patsy caught her breath and I struggled for composure. There Trevor was, lying in a surgical bed, hooked up to an IV, an oxygen mask on his face, with two chest tubes sticking out from his tiny ribs, hooked up to suction drainage. He recognized us, but our usually articulate son didn't say anything. Not a word. He didn't even cry. I'm sure he hadn't the foggiest idea what had happened to him — why he hurt so much. He was just lying there, stunned. I had seen hundreds of children postoperatively, *but they hadn't been mine!*

Trevor was in the hospital for about a week. I canceled my entire surgical schedule, and Patsy and I spent every moment allowed with him. Within two days the chest tubes and the IV were out and he was eating. Tests showed that the remaining upper lobe of the right lung had expanded satisfactorily. He proved to be the center of attention because he was such a beautiful little boy with a bubbly disposition and a pleasant smile. Because of that — and maybe because they knew he was mine — the nurses gave him more attention than was necessary. It's funny how some of the little things stand out. Since he was forced to lie on his back for a number of days, he developed the habit of crossing one foot over the knee of his other leg to be more comfortable — but it's a position that children usually don't assume; it's an adult idiosyncrasy — and he looked quite comical.

Once Trevor was discharged from the hospital, he continued to do well at home. And then the multiple conferences began with the Pediatric Hematology Department to determine what further therapy was necessary. X-ray treatments were discussed, but it was decided that they were unnecessary, since the tumor apparently had been completely removed. Instead, to avoid any possible recurrence, one full year of chemotherapy was recommended. It was unanimously agreed that he be started on a program called VAC, in which three chemotherapeutic drugs — vincristine, actinomycin, and Cytoxan — would be given by needle every day for a period of one week. Then five weeks would be skipped, and the treatment would be repeated, until fifty-two weeks had passed. Although some facilities insist that the patient be admitted during the drug or "pulse" weeks, our Pediatric Department's policy was that the patient did better at home, with hospitalization only if necessary.

There is no denying that chemotherapy is a miserable thing to go through. The idea is that the drugs will kill any cancer cells because they have a high metabolic rate — they are rapidly reproducing and therefore are susceptible to being killed off. However, chemotherapy is not without major side effects. One is that it knocks the white cell count down to dangerous levels — so low that if an infection occurs during that period, it can become life-threatening. The body's resistance has, in essence, been eliminated.

Trevor got into serious trouble within ten days of his first treatment. One of the drugs gave him an intestinal ileus — a distended bowel that would not function. We rushed him to the hospital. There a test indicated that his white blood cell count had plummeted down to eighty-five granulocytes. (Granulocytes are three of the five types of white blood cells and the most significant in fighting infection. The normal count is in the range of three thousand five hundred.) Then Trevor developed a fever.

No one kidded anybody. It was a critical situation. His best chance for survival was a white cell transfusion. I would be the donor. The only problem was that the equipment needed was so sophisticated, costly, and rare that it was available only in certain centers throughout the country. So we frantically made plans for an emergency air flight to Stanford Medical Center. Long distance calls sped back and forth. Arrangements were made. We would leave the next morning.

That evening I helped Patsy pack. The horrifying thought was present in both our minds. Three of us were going. Would three be returning — or only two? Later that night we rushed back to the hospital. Miracle of miracles, Trevor's white cell count had started to rise, and we were able to cancel our plans for the time being. Finally the distension of his abdomen relented. Once again we were able to take Trevor home.

It was a couple of weeks before his hair began to fall

out — another side effect of the chemotherapy. As I've mentioned, our cat Marmalade was an Angora. In happier times, when Patsy would pick tufts of shed hair from the floor, she would hold them up to Trevor and, with a wry grin, explain, "Kitty-cat!" The first time Trevor ran his hands through his hair, a large patch came out and stuck to his little fingers. With a wide, knowledgeable grin, he ran to Patsy.

"Kitty-cat!" he chuckled gleefully. "Kitty-cat!"

Within three weeks, Trevor was completely bald. With all our other problems, it seems odd to say that it was one of the hardest things to bear. Perhaps it was because it was a constant reminder of the deadly cloud hanging over us. A month before, we'd had a beautiful little boy with blond curly hair. Now we had a bald child who was terribly sick and who'd lost so much weight you could scarcely find him in his clothes.

Patsy searched out a seamstress and had a whole wardrobe of little hats made for him with bands attached so they couldn't fall off. It was difficult to let him out of our sight, but we gritted our teeth and started him in a local Montessori school, determined that he have the opportunity to socialize with other children as much as he could during the periods when he was feeling well. It didn't matter that he missed about half of the school sessions; at least he had contact with kids his own age.

Inside or out, Trevor *always* wore his hat. It became accepted and, surprisingly, very little was made of it at the school. It was funny, but there was another little boy in class who loved a particular cap he owned and insisted on wearing it constantly. There was nothing wrong with him — he had a full head of hair — he just liked that hat! So, as far as the other children were concerned, Trevor wasn't any different from that little boy. It was always our fear that he would be subjected to ridicule by his schoolmates, or that his hat would fall off while playing. I guess we were supersensitive about this, for it was no great problem.

Except once. It was a hot day and Patsy was shopping with our son at the local supermarket. As she was going through the checkout line, the cashier spied Trevor.

"My, what a cute little boy. How come you're wearing a hat? Aren't you warm? Let's see what color hair you have —"

Even as she reached out, Patsy screamed, *"Don't!* Leave him alone!" Too late. The checkout girl's face turned beet-red and she apologized profusely. Patsy was furious, even though she realized the girl's intentions and motives were the best. And Trevor? It didn't bother him in the least.

Meanwhile the drug therapy continued every sixth week. For fourteen days after that, Trevor's white cell count would again become dangerously low. We had to watch him like a pair of hawks during that time, checking him constantly for fever. When the two weeks were up, he was relatively safe again, but I lost track of the countless times we rushed him to the hospital to be checked and started on antibiotics.

We had adjusted pretty well — and then the wheezing attacks began. At first we thought it was related to his loss of lung tissue through surgery, but then it was determined that Trevor was an asthmatic! It was almost too much. The attacks would occur at anytime, often in the middle of the night, and we'd rush him into the hospital for epinephrine shots at the Emergency Room. The thing we feared most was that Trevor would have an asthma attack during a period when his resistance was at its lowest. Miraculously, that never happened.

Throughout all this, Patsy was heroic. Only once did she break. She was eight and a half months pregnant. I was in my office when I got a call from the pediatrician's nurse, who said that Patsy was there with Trevor and was very upset. Panicked, I raced over and, for the first time, found her in tears. Trevor had become sick and had thrown up all over the car; then as she was turning into the hospital, she'd been involved in a minor auto accident. I guess the combination was just too much. But even as I began to comfort her, she regained her composure and was off to get Trevor his treatment. It was she, much more than I, who bore the brunt of responsibility for caring for our son during that time, and she did a marvelous job: Trevor, in spite of everything, is tremendously well adjusted and bears no psychological scars from his ordeal. Patsy made it a point to buy countless children's hospital books and read them to him, illustrating the point that lots of kids go through medical experiences. We got doctor kits and he had a little boy-doll that he dearly loved. He'd carefully wrap the tourniquet, put a needle into boy-doll, and give him his medicine. Trevor looked upon the whole thing as some kind of game. I estimate that he had, in all, more than five hundred injections. He got to the point where he would tell the doctor where he wanted the shot.

Even when Tyler, our second son was born, Patsy managed. I don't know how — but she managed.

Every three months Trevor had chest X-rays, and I was always with him. He got to be a total professional, knowing just how to stand, in exactly what position to turn. Every three months I would look at those chest X-rays, holding my breath, praying that there'd be no abnormality. And run to call Patsy with the good news.

And then I had to call her with bad news. As the year was nearing its end — just as we felt the chemotherapy ordeal might be over — the pediatrician readjusted his recommendation — and another full year of treatment was ordered.

It's strange. Early on, we had actually psyched ourselves into realizing that Trevor might die. We were biding our time. Toward the end of the second year, however, we began to appreciate that his chances were really pretty good, what with the complete surgical removal of the tumor and twenty-four months of prophylactic chemotherapy, we were quoted statistics that the odds were ninety percent he'd be okay — and every day the odds got better.

The treatments have been discontinued now. The

weight loss has been regained; his curly blond hair has grown back. He does occasionally ask why he has that large scar on his chest, and we try to answer within the range of his understanding.

It was hard. But it made me a better human being. And a better doctor. I bleed for my patients. I know what their loved ones are going through. I thought I did before — but I didn't. Until you've gone through the experience yourself, you only kid yourself by saying you understand.

Chapter Seventeen

M Y PLASTIC SURGERY RESIDENCY at University
Hospital would be coming to an end in about
two months, and it was time for a series of momentous
decisions.

Where to set up my private practice? That was the
biggest question of all, for along with career and financial considerations, it would also dictate where we
would live — probably for the rest of our lives. Patsy
and I gave it a great deal of thought and discussed it
for hours on end. We finally approached it backward —
where did we want to live? We ended up making a list
of things most important to us. At the very top was
what location would be best for the children, especially
for Trevor, for we were determined that he should
have an easy ride for a while. We wanted a good climate, where the pace was less hectic than in this city,
and one that had a low crime rate. There had to be
easy access to the things little boys like to do. The city

couldn't be too big or too small, and it should offer an above-average quality of life. We came up with and rejected a dozen cities before we zeroed in on one. San Diego.

It had a lot going for it. It had the best climate in the country. It had beaches, and Sea World, and the zoo, and one of the best wild animal parks in the world. It was also in Southern California, and I knew I would get referrals from past patients. Many cosmetic surgery patients prefer to have their operation away from home, away from prying eyes and questioning friends. At the same time, they'd want a warm, pleasant, leisurely atmosphere. San Diego could offer that.

Patsy and I wore a path between home and San Diego, exploring the possibilities. We were drawn to a suburb about thirteen miles north of the heart of San Diego. Being a New Englander, I like trees. Palms were okay, but I missed the oaks and elms. Even though most of San Diego has a desert-like terrain similar to Mexico's, this area was hilly and abounded with beautiful eucalyptus trees that rustled and swayed and emitted a delightful aroma. Patsy and I knew we could be happy here.

We found a house for sale in an area that was part of a planned community. There were a swimming pool and six tennis courts — and Patsy and I were tennis freaks. Most important, there was a marvelous children's play area with sandboxes, slides, swings, and toy rocking horses. Where there are playgrounds, there are lots of other kids, and we knew Trevor and Tyler would have a ball. There were planned luaus and pot-luck dinners, which would be great for meeting our neighbors and making new friends. As a dedicated jog-ger, I noticed that the streets were wide and traffic was light.

The house we were most taken with was on a dead-end street, which offered a fairly safe play area for children, and so many kids lived there that they were self-entertaining. Most had little plastic tricycles with Batman images all over them. Watching, Trevor was entranced. All the way home, he prattled about his very own Batcycle: what color he wanted, where he would garage it, and whether he'd take Tyler for a ride.

We wanted that house badly, but caution was the watchword. A quick check indicated there were al-ready over thirty plastic surgeons practicing in San Diego. From a competitive standpoint, it was probably the worst city in the country, except for San Francisco, for an ambitious young plastic surgeon to get his start.

And that brought me to question number two. I had already decided that the ideal arrangement for starting private practice would be an expense-sharing arrange-ment with an already established doctor. It's rather startling to think of, but it costs at least seventy thou-sand dollars to open and equip your own office. An ophthalmologist friend of mine had taken that route about five years before. Besides the sizable monthly payment on his loan, he was faced with a thousand-dollar-a-month rent, plus salaries, equipment, and in-surance. Although he'd envisioned a rosy future, when

I'd last spoken to him, he'd admitted he was barely eking out a living. I had no intention of digging a similar hole for myself and spending the next decade trying to climb out of it. So, I would sublease an office from another physician. But with whom? Luckily, again I sought out the advice of friends and colleagues who'd been through the experience.

A friend of mine, Dr. Joseph Wall, also a plastic surgeon, was practicing in a nearby city. He'd been a little ahead of me in training and had encountered the problems of entering private practice about a year before. In talking to him, I got the benefit of some eye-opening inside advice. Joe had also seen the wisdom of sharing expenses and had made arrangements to subrent space from a Dr. Abbott, who was a considerably older and well-known plastic surgeon. Joe immediately ran into scheduling problems. Although the senior doctor tried to cooperate, my friend found himself with last pick on operating room time and office hours.

There was another conflict, too. Dr. Abbott did considerable trauma work, while Joe specialized in cosmetic cases. Frequently in the communal waiting room, there would be several well-dressed, affluent ladies waiting for a consultation with Dr. Wall. Sitting in opposite chairs would be a couple of motorcycle riders who'd injured themselves trying to commit what we rather sarcastically call "Honda-cide." From scraping along the road, they had all sorts of horrible bruises and deformities and sutured lacerations.

Then Joe became aware of another problem. Patients would call and ask: "Which of the doctors is the best?" The reply was that both were fully trained and competent. But then they'd ask which had the most experience, and the honest answer was that Dr. Abbott had been practicing for twenty years, and Dr. Wall had been practicing for two. You can imagine the result. For a while my friend believed that it would work in his favor to have his fees about half of those charged by Abbott. Wrong. For some reason, prospective patients figured if the one man charged twice as much as the other, he had to be twice as good. There was also the problem of patients comparing notes. No two doctors' techniques are the same. Neither one is right or wrong — they just operate differently. This the patients couldn't understand, and it left them uneasy and unsure.

Taking my friend's experiences to heart, I decided I'd be better off sharing facilities with a general surgeon who would not be competitive in my own field. As luck would have it, I was able to find a young general surgeon who was as anxious as I was for such an arrangement. His offices were modern and well equipped, with a minor operating room, which suited me to a T. Best of all, our building housed many doctors, none of whom were plastic surgeons. The possibility of patient referrals from them would be a big plus. And the final asset that made up my mind: adjoining was a small but very fine private hospital with top-notch facilities — and with no staff plastic surgeon.

Everything fell into place. We closed the escrow on

our dream house and I entered into a sublease arrangement for office space. Luckily, banks consider doctors pretty good risks, for besides the house and additional furniture, a big expense was buying my own surgical instruments. There is a vast variety available, and I had my pets. More than that, I wanted the best.

So now we had a house — and I had an office. The only thing missing was prospective patients. It's something every young doctor faces — how to start and build up his practice. As I've mentioned, I knew I would draw referrals from my former University Hospital patients. Oddly enough, about eighty percent of a plastic surgeon's practice is made up of friends and relatives of pleased ex-patients. I agreed to lecture at women's clubs and, to my delight, found myself greatly in demand. Plastic surgery is a subject of widespread interest, and before long I knew that many members of the audiences would be seeking me out. I contacted the emergency rooms at the various San Diego hospitals and told them I was available. Two or three cases a week of that type would pay the rent.

I knew that every decision had been solidly made. Yet the thought of leaving the cocoon of University Hospital, which had been my base of operations for so long, was scary.

On my last day at the hospital I didn't expect bands or a farewell party or any great show of emotions. People came and people went in a large medical center. There were ongoing problems and a routine to be followed. Nevertheless, I was a little surprised that the day I left was pretty much like any other day. I made morning rounds with Dr. Parmenter and Dr. Burke. When we'd finished, Parmenter slapped me on the shoulder.

"Don, it's been good. As far as I'm concerned, you'll always be my number one resident. Best of luck. Keep in touch." And he was off.

Burke stared at me, almost enviously. "Let me know how it goes," he muttered. "I hear it's a jungle out there."

I didn't expect a nostalgic or prolonged farewell from Miss Farrell, and she was right in character when she merely nodded her good-bye and checked to make sure I had left behind the department's medical dictionary and anatomy study skull.

I wandered down to Emergency — but three patients were brought in almost simultaneously. The nurses there were flying.

"It's been nice working with you, Dr. Moynihan."

"Good luck."

It was all there was time for.

I said good-bye to the floor and surgical nurses. And made it a point to thank all the technicians in X-ray and in the lab who'd been so kind. To Trevor. To Patsy. To me.

And then, not knowing what else to do, I slowly headed for the parking lot.

I was excited about the challenge of private practice. There was a horde of people out there with problems and deformities I could help. And I would, too. I was looking forward to it. But I'd miss University Hospital. The years I had spent there had been wonderful ones. So much had happened.

Now I was leaving for the last time. I looked back at the hospital. Then up at the sky. Shouldn't the sun go in, or something? Maybe an earthquake — just a little one? Something — anything — to announce the making of a plastic surgeon?